I0222600

ACID REFLUX DIET

How to Adopt an Effettive Acid Reflux Diet to Stop Your
Heartburn Problems

(Paleo and Gluten-free Recipes to Manage and Relief Reflux)

David Montgomery

Published by Alex Howard

© **David Montgomery**

All Rights Reserved

Acid Reflux Diet: How to Adopt an Effettive Acid Reflux Diet to Stop Your Heartburn Problems (Paleo and Gluten-free Recipes to Manage and Relief Reflux)

ISBN 978-1-77485-004-6

All rights reserved. No part of this guide may be reproduced in any form without permission in writing from the publisher except in the case of brief quotations embodied in critical articles or reviews.

Legal & Disclaimer

The information contained in this book is not designed to replace or take the place of any form of medicine or professional medical advice. The information in this book has been provided for educational and entertainment purposes only.

The information contained in this book has been compiled from sources deemed reliable, and it is accurate to the best of the Author's knowledge; however, the Author cannot guarantee its accuracy and validity and cannot be held liable for any errors or omissions. Changes are periodically made to this book. You must consult your doctor or get professional medical advice before using any of the suggested remedies, techniques, or information in this book.

Table of contents

Part 1

Chapter 1: What is acid reflux disease: Introduction

Sixty percent of the adult population will experience some form of GERD or Acid Reflux within any given twelve-month period of time. It is estimated that over twenty percent of the U.S. population experience Acid Reflux symptoms at least weekly. Even children under the age of seventeen are experiencing a dramatic increase in the number of them that are suffering from the effects of reflux. So what is Acid Reflux and GERD? Who get it? And what causes it?

Most people have experienced the typical burning sensation in the chest that often occurs after eating a meal. The most common reason for this symptom is an increased production of stomach acid. However, there is another common reason for this symptom. It is known as the regurgitation of food from the stomach to the esophagus. Typically, after eructation a person will experience a strong burning and irritating sensation in the throat. This is the typical symptom of the regurgitative disorder called Acid Reflux Disease.

Acid reflux, which is quite common in western populations, is the burning sensation in the lower chest that occurs when the acidic contents of the stomach flow back into the food pipe or the esophagus. If it occurs frequently, it is called gastroesophageal reflux disease (GERD). Acid reflux is also called heartburn or acid indigestion. It usually occurs after a heavy meal.

The strong hydrochloric acid produced by the stomach lining promotes food digestion and eliminates harmful bacteria. The lining also protects the stomach from the effects of the acid. The esophagus does not have such a protective lining. It is protected by the gastroesophageal sphincter, a ring of muscles, which act as a one-way valve allowing food to pass into the stomach, but blocking anything that tries to come back thru to the esophagus. When this mechanism fails to operate properly, the acidic contents of the stomach can go back into the esophagus, resulting in a burning sensation.

The typical symptoms of acid reflux are:

- Heartburn, which is an uncomfortable burning sensation in the esophagus, usually felt behind the breastbone. It may originate in the abdomen and spread to the neck or the throat. It can aggravate you when you lie down or bend over. It can last for up to two hours and gets worse after eating.
- Regurgitation of the bitter acidic fluid into the mouth that leaves a bitter taste and a burning sensation in the mouth.
- Sore throat and trouble in swallowing.
- Persistent dry cough.

- Hoarseness in the morning.
- Wheezing and nausea.
- Children and infants may vomit, cough and have respiratory problems.
- Bad breath.

People of all ages can be affected by recurring acid reflux. There are various factors that can contribute to the development of this condition. One such factor is a physical abnormality called a hiatus hernia. It consists of a hole in the diaphragm that allows a part of the stomach to enter the chest cavity and cause GERD. Pregnancy can also lead to acid reflux because there is additional pressure on the internal organs. The other factors that can contribute to the development of GERD involve lifestyle or dietary issues. Although all the reasons for the occurrence of acid reflux are not known, it can typically be blamed on various lifestyle choices or conditions such as:

- High salt intake
- Obesity
- Low intake of dietary fiber
- Active or passive smoking
- Absence of sufficient exercise
- Intake of drugs for asthma, painkillers, antidepressants, sedatives and antihistamines

It is wise not to leave acid reflux or GERD untreated for prolong periods of time. If left untreated, it can lead to many complications, some of which can be very serious. They include:

- An increased risk of cancer. Frequent heartburn can be a precursor to cancer of the esophagus or the vocal cord.
- Inflammation of the esophagus lining causes irritation, bleeding or even ulcer formation.
- Repeated ulceration of the esophageal tissues lead to the formation of a scar, which has no elasticity. As a result, a stricture (an abnormal narrowing or contraction of a body passage or opening) is formed that lacks the ability to expand and relax to facilitate the passage of food through the esophagus. Due to this, food tends to get stuck at different places in the esophagus as it moves down towards the stomach.
- The acid damage produces a scar that makes swallowing difficult.
- In Barrett's esophagus, the tissue lining the esophagus changes into those similar to the cells in the lower gastrointestinal tract. These cells have a higher tendency of turning malignant.

There are some simple things that can help acid reflux symptoms diminish be done away with completely.

These include: the avoidance of food, drink and medication that can be linked to your heartburn, eating smaller meals, avoiding lying down for two to three hours after a meal, losing weight (if you are even slightly obese), avoiding increased pressure on your abdomen for any reason and stop smoking.

The first thing a person affected by acid reflux should do is to keep a diary of, and carefully describe in detail, the circumstances that led to the symptoms of acid reflux including: the food, drink, smoking, medication or stress that may have caused it. Everything should be written down and accounted for in the diary. It should be studied to find out the correlation between the heartburns and the particular trigger. Avoidance of such triggers should decrease the frequency of the attacks.

If these lifestyle changes do not lead to relief of the symptoms and their frequency, you should consult a doctor who may advise you of tests and subsequent treatment with various drugs that can alleviate the acid reflux. However, most patients obtain substantial relief by following a well planned diet and making some simple changes in their lifestyle. The next chapters are focused on providing some simple tricks to help control acid reflux and to manage the disease effectively thus improving your quality of life.

Chapter 2: The recommended GERD Diet for patients with Acid reflux disease

The lower end of the esophagus has a ring of muscles that acts as a one-way gate for the food to pass thru to the stomach. It then stops anything from returning from the stomach back into the food pipe. When its operation becomes faulty, the acidic contents of the stomach splash back into the esophagus, creating heartburn. Hoarseness, cough and shortness of breath can also occur when the stomach's contents seep back into the breathing tubes. As discussed earlier, this problem is called Gastroesophageal Reflux Disease (GERD).

Cereals, vegetables, fruits, dairy products and meats are usually safe and do not lead to GERD. However, there are certain types of food that can contribute to the relaxation of the lower esophageal muscle, thus causing GERD.

If someone cannot tolerate oranges or tomato due to their acidic nature, a vitamin C supplement becomes necessary. Listed below are some foods that can aggravate GERD symptoms and should be removed from the diet of a person suffering from it:

- Fatty or fried food
- Whole milk
- Food or soup made with cream
- Fast food
- Peppermint and spearmint
- Oils
- Chocolate
- Onions
- Alcohol
- Stop consuming tobacco in all forms because nicotine weakens the esophageal muscles
- Shun chewing gum and hard candy as they lead to the swallowing of more air, which causes belching and reflux. (As discussed, later chewing gum can possibly help with acid reflux in certain individuals and situations. Gum chewing is something that can be tried, with the effect noted, to determine if it should be continued or stopped.)

Some foods cause irritation and inflammation of the lower esophagus and their intake has to be curtailed or avoided altogether. Here is a list of such foods:

- Citrus fruits like grapefruit, orange, pineapple, tomato and their juice
- Coffee
- Caffeinated soft drinks
- Tea
- Spicy or acidic food

An important aspect of a GERD diet is that some foods in some groups can be eaten, while others in the same group have to be avoided.

Low-fat milk can be consumed, while whole milk and chocolate milk should be avoided. While most vegetables can be consumed, fried or creamy vegetables and tomatoes must be avoided. While apples, bananas, pears, melons, peaches and berries can be included in the diet; oranges, grapefruit and pineapple should not be. Breads and grains with low-fat content are okay; but not those prepared with whole milk or high-fat.

Meat, chicken, fish and turkey are fine; but cold cuts, bacon, sausage, chicken fat and skin and fatty meat are on the banned list. Sweets made with low or no fat are allowed, but chocolate and desserts made with oils and fats are not. Soups too should be fat-free or low-fat based.

Then there are some GERD-friendly foods that can help patients reduce their symptoms. These are:

- Yogurt contains good bacteria called probiotics. They promote digestion and offer some protection against harmful bacteria. Probiotics can be helpful for most people suffering from GERD.
- An increased fiber intake from fruits and vegetables is helpful against GERD, although no one is sure

exactly how it works. Increasing dietary fiber though is a prove wise step.

- Lean proteins are highly recommended for GERD patients. Eggs an example of food high in protein. If eggs in general cause a problem, try only the egg white by removing the yolk.
- Opt for grilled, poached, broiled or baked lean meats.
- Complex carbohydrates from oatmeal, whole grain bread, rice, and couscous should form a large chunk of your daily diet.
- Potatoes and other root vegetables are good sources of healthy carbs and digestible fiber.
- Consume unsaturated fats from plants or fish like olive, canola, avocados, sesame, sunflower, peanuts and peanut butter. Polyunsaturated fats like safflower, soybean and corn, and fatty fish like salmon and trout are also excellent.

However, since individuals differ greatly in their response to various types of foods, some people may not be affected at all by the foods listed here that are known to aggravate the GERD symptoms, while others may have a negative reaction to the healthy and safe foods listed here. GERD patients have to modify these lists to fit themselves and manage their diet in order to achieve the best results. This can best be done by maintaining a diary of what you eat, when you eat, how much you eat and what is the result.

If there is any doubt about a certain food, you can try it in less quantity initially, and then gradually increase the amount you consume until you reach the amount a normal person would consume in order to see if you develop any symptoms. This will help you create a list of foods that are healthy, safe, balanced, varied and enjoyable.

Chapter 3: Awesome recipes that can help control the symptoms of GERD (including links to over 200 recipes)

GERD is the result of the acidic contents in the stomach splashing back into the esophagus because of the malfunctioning of the ring of muscles at the lower end of the esophagus. If the acidic contents of the stomach leak into the wind pipe, it can also cause sore throat, trouble in swallowing, persistent dry cough and hoarseness. Diet has a considerable bearing on the incidence of GERD symptoms. Here are some GERD-friendly recipes you might want to try:

1. Green bean casserole

This is a great tasting casserole that can be prepared in a short period of time. It is also easy to prepare. It might also go well with leftover chicken or turkey meat. All its ingredients are usually available in the kitchen. It can also be reheated, if necessary. It is as tasty as it is nutritious. Many people with and without GERD symptoms are sure to love it. Here is how to make it:

The ingredients are: 1 can of reduced-fat cream mushroom soup, 2 cups frozen green beans, 1-3/4 cups uncooked egg noodles, 1/4th cup no-fat sour cream, 1 cup water, 1/4th cup low-fat cheddar cheese, 1-1/2 diced chicken or turkey meat, $1/4^{th}$ teaspoon turmeric and $1/4^{th}$ teaspoon black pepper.

Mix the mushroom soup and water in a large skillet and add the green beans, uncooked noodles and chicken meat. Cook for about 15 minutes, stirring occasionally until the noodles become tender. Add seasonings, sour cream and cheddar cheese. Allow the mix to simmer for 5 minutes until the cheese melts.

2. Apple pie-pork chops

This recipe has been compared to warm apple pie. Its ingredients are: 1 tablespoon canola oil, 4 pork loin chops, 1 tablespoon soft margarine, 1/2 teaspoon ground cinnamon, 3 tablespoons brown sugar, 1/4 teaspoon ground nutmeg, 3 peeled and chopped apples, 3 tablespoon chopped walnuts and 1 tablespoon apple juice.

Mix brown sugar, cinnamon and nutmeg. Heat oil in a skillet and add pork chops. Cook each side for 3 or 4 minutes. Set them aside. Then put the butter and brown sugar mixture into a pan. Cook on low heat for half a minute. Add the apples and apple juice and stir for a few minutes until the apples turn soft. Put the pork chops back into the pan, turn and let them soak up the apple flavor. Top the pork chops with the apple mixture and serve.

3. Shrimp stir fry

This recipe is another one that can be prepared rather quickly if you are in a hurry. Fresh shrimp, cabbage, sweet bell pepper and frozen peas are used here. Season the mix with ginger.

The ingredients are: 2 tablespoons finely grated ginger, 1 chopped sweet bell pepper, 1 tablespoon olive oil, 2/3rd pound sliced white cabbage, 4 tablespoons chopped cilantro, 1 teaspoon sesame oil, 3/4 pound cooked and peeled shrimp and 1-1/2 cups frozen peas.

Heat the oil. Stir-fry ginger and chopped bell pepper for one minute. Add peas. Stir-fry for 2 minutes. Add cabbage and stir-fry for 2 to 3 minutes. Add shrimp and cook until it is cooked through (until pink on all sides) for approximately one minute. Stir in the cilantro and serve.

4. Quick banana sorbet

This is a nice dish for hot days and it is also quite easy to make. The ingredients are 3 peeled bananas, 3 cups ice, 1 tablespoon finely grated ginger, 1/8 teaspoon ground cardamom, ¼ teaspoon salt and 2 tablespoon honey.

Blend bananas, ginger, cardamom, honey and salt into a smooth mix. Add ice and continue blending to make the mix creamy. Serve immediately or store in the freezer.

5. Oatmeal

This is a good breakfast dish, that is a healthy to eat and very easy to make. The ingredients are: 1 cup instant oatmeal, 2 tablespoon raisins, 1 cup (non or low fat milk), ½ peeled and diced golden apple, ½ diced banana, 2 teaspoon honey and a pinch of salt.

Mix oatmeal, milk, raisins, salt and honey the evening before if possible or at least three hours before making the dish. Place the mix in the refrigerator. When ready to eat, cook mixture thoroughly. Add fruits before serving. Add (non or low fat) milk, if necessary.

Chapter 4: Effective natural herbs and home remedies for treating Acid Reflux

There are a number of chemical-based medications that claim to offer immediate relief to people suffering from heartburn and acid reflux. However, the relief provided by the over-the-counter and prescription medicines is often only temporary.

On the other hand, some people prefer adopting lifestyle changes that will help them overcome the burning sensation caused by acid reflux permanently. One such change includes the use of herbal remedies, that can easily be prepared at home.

In a later chapter we will examine some of the lifestyle changes that can help a patient treat and avoid acid reflux. Now though, we will discuss some of the best herbs and simple home remedies that can be used to treat acid reflux:

Mustard

Mustard is highly alkaline in nature, making it a wonderful remedy to help balance the acidity caused by acid reflux. It may seem a bit odd to ingest mustard directly as first but give it a try. Many patients say that it does wonders when it comes to the treatment of acid reflux.

Mustard acts as one of the most wonderful remedies for most stomach ailments including acid reflux. Therefore, don't hesitate to pop some mustard in the middle of a heartburn flare-up or when you feel like you are about to have one.

Apple Cider Vinegar

One of the common misunderstandings associated with acid reflux is that it is caused only by the presence of an excessive amount of acid in the stomach. This myth has become prevalent thanks to the presence of "acid blockers" in the commonly available over-the-counter medications for heartburn.

However, the presence of too little acid in the stomach may also cause acid reflux. The higher amount of acid in the stomach secreted in response to the food you have eaten tells the lower esophageal sphincter (LES) to close off so that there is no movement of the acid from the stomach to the esophagus. In the absence of an adequate amount of acid in the stomach, the LES loosens up a bit and this can result in the acid reflux.

Therefore, sometimes consuming more acid can help curb acid reflux. Apple cider vinegar is one such remedy that can rescue you if this is the case.

Try consuming 1 tablespoon of apple cider vinegar diluted in six to eight ounces of water to obtain quick relief from the symptoms.

Aloe Juice

Aloe juice is known to provide relief in cases of severe burns, sunburn and inflammation. The soothing property of aloe vera is not restricted just to the external parts of the body; it can also help to ease and soothe the digestive tract.

The anti-inflammatory action of aloe vera juice can help treat heartburn. When you feel that your stomach or esophagus is irritated because of acid reflux, try consuming a glass of fresh aloe vera juice to get rid of the condition instantly. Regular consumption of this juice will prevent the inflammation around the lower esophageal region and reduce the risk of ulcers and cancer.

Another tasty way to consume aloe vera is with products like aloe vera water. A favorite among many people is aloe vera water mixed with mango. It provides a tasty sweet healthy drink. This water can be found by using the following link: **aloe vera water with mango.**

Sodium Bicarbonate

Sodium bicarbonate, commonly known as baking soda, also acts as an excellent home remedy when it comes to the burning sensation caused by the acid reflux. Sodium bicarbonate is basic in nature. Therefore, it helps neutralize the acid present in the stomach. So if the LES decides to loosen up a bit, sodium bicarbonate makes sure that the acid reaching your throat is neutralized, thereby sparing you of any burning sensation.

Banana/Apple

Bananas contain antacids that help balance the acid. The simplest herbal remedy to treat heartburn and acid reflux is to consume one fully-ripened banana every day. You may even try slicing up an apple every day and consuming it during the day or better yet, a few hours before laying down to sleep at night.

Chewing Gum

A research conducted by The Journal of Dental Research showed that chewing gum can help provide relief to people with chronic heartburn and GERD. During the study, the participants were asked to chew a piece of sugar-free gum for 30 minutes after a meal.

Chewing gum triggers the salivary glands to produce more saliva. The excessive amount of saliva dilutes the acid that reaches up into the throat and thus neutralizes and washes it away. This helps to provide relief from GERD symptoms.

Other than the aforementioned remedies, you can also try consuming a cup of mint, fenugreek or chamomile tea. Health experts advise people prone to heartburn to pop in three to four raw almonds after every meal to eliminate the risk of a burning sensation caused by the acid reflux. Almonds help balance the pH in the stomach.

In this chapter, we examined some of the easiest herbal remedies that you can quickly use in case of mild to moderate acid reflux. It costs very little to try these remedies before you decide to get temporary relief by means of over-the-counter pills and prescription medication.

Chapter 5: Modern Medical Solutions that can provide relief from Acid Reflux

By making simple changes in your diet and lifestyle, you can successfully manage the symptoms of acid reflux. Although these things are effective at helping you deal with the occasional bouts of acid reflux, you may need to take medication, especially if you are suffering from severe symptoms associated with acid reflux.

In this section, you will find some modern solutions for acid reflux, which can provide instant relief from the symptoms. If ignored, the disease may become severe and in the end may require you to have surgery.

Medication used to combat acid reflux

Typically, doctors will recommend that you start medications if you have the symptoms on a daily basis or more than three times a week. Listed below are some of the most effective medicines used to treat acid reflux:

- **Oral suspension medications** are frequently used to treat acid reflux and other associated symptoms

25

such as diarrhea, nausea, stomach ulcers, throat ulcers and intestine ulcers. These liquid suspensions form a protective layer on the inner side of the esophagus and protect it from the damage caused by gastric acid.

- **Antacids** neutralize the excess stomach acid and provide immediate relief in mild to moderate cases of acid reflux. Several antacids are available in liquid form that cover the inner wall of the esophagus and reduce the production of stomach acid. Though antacids are not helpful in reducing inflammation associated with acid reflux, it is a good option for obtaining quick relief from severe heartburn.

- **Proton pump inhibitors or PPIs** are another effective treatment. These medications act by blocking the acid production in the stomach and assist in healing the inner wall of the esophagus. If you are suffering from more frequent and severe symptoms of acid reflux, proton pump inhibitors can help you. Some PPIs are available as OTC medicines, while others should only be taken under medical supervision. PPIs are considered a standard treatment for acid reflux as they are absolutely safe and cause minimal side effects.

- **H2 receptor blockers** are over-the-counter medicines that act by curbing the acid production in the stomach. It is used to treat mild cases of acid reflux. Although it lacks the quick relief action provided by the antacids, being inexpensive and their ability to provide a longer-lasting relief than the antacids, make them a popular medication to treat acid reflux.

When is a surgery required?

If medication doesn't stop your acid reflux, the resulting prolonged exposure of the esophageal mucosa to the gastric acid may lead to severe complications of GERD such as erosive esophagitis, Barrett's esophagus, esophageal stricture, aspiration pneumonia and adenocarcinoma. Surgical treatment for GERD is recommended for treating chronic situations.

If you are suffering from extremely severe symptoms associated with acid reflux, then surgery is a good option to the prolonged medical therapy. To treat severe and complicated acid reflux, it is advisable to opt for surgery because it offers better and faster results compared to the medical therapy.

The surgery corrects the undetected causes of GERD. Apart from this, it also repairs the hiatal hernia and improves the gastric emptying and the esophageal motility. It can also help to elongate the lower esophageal sphincter. It creates a preventive barrier that prevents the damages from the acid reflux as well as from the bile reflux and the regurgitation of food. These advantages make surgery a more effective option for curbing the symptoms and the progression of acid reflux to its more serious form.

The most widely-performed surgical procedure for GERD is known as fundoplication or Nissen fundoplication.

A minimally invasive technique called Laparoscopic surgery is the gold standard for surgical treatment of severe GERD. Laparoscopic surgery has advantages over Nissen fundoplication.

It is important to carefully select over-the-counter medications as some of them may cause a few side effects. Patients are advised to take the medications under the supervision of a physician.

While modern medical therapy seems to be extremely effective in curbing acid reflux symptoms, the surgical therapy has been significantly more beneficial as the continuous use of medications may cause relapses and progression of the disease if the patient does not follow the dietary and lifestyle recommendations mentioned in the previous chapters.

Chapter 6: Tips to Get Rid of Acid Reflux Forever

Acid reflux is a major concern for many people. If you have it, you undoubtedly have experienced severe heartburn at one point or another. Some have acid reflux symptoms once or twice a month. Others more frequently. It is neither possible nor is it safe to have antacids every time you have a bout of acid reflux. On the other hand, an untreated and continuous acid reflux issue can lead to severe consequences like esophageal cancer. This is because heartburn or acid reflux is the result of stomach acids streaming back into the esophagus. This can corrode and damage the delicate esophageal mucosa.

So how can this problem be resolved permanently? Well, worry no more! Here are some great tips and remedies that can help you rid yourself of acid reflux forever.

Get Rid of Acid Reflux

Midnight acid reflux creates a level of discomfort and the resulting bitter taste can not only disturb your sleep, but even make it elusive. If you are looking for a way to treat acid reflux permanently, you are advised to make some changes in your lifestyle as well as in your diet. Here are some helpful tips that will enable you to do just that:

- **Maintain a healthy weight**

Even the slightest increase in your weight can worsen heartburn symptoms. Maintaining a healthy body weight can help you reduce the symptoms of acid reflux.

- **Wear loose fit clothes**

Tight clothes, specifically around the waist, can put pressure on the stomach. This can result in an aggravation of the acid reflux symptoms. Therefore, make sure you wear loose-fitting clothes, especially around the waist and when going to bed.

- **Avoid trigger foods**

Make a note of the foods that trigger acid reflux. These foods can be different for each person. The common foods known to cause exacerbations include: onions, garlic, peppermint, caffeinated drinks, chocolate, fatty foods and spicy or fried foods. Additionally, citrus fruits like oranges can also cause acid reflux.

- **Relax while you eat**

Stressful eating or eating in a hurry can cause a higher production of the acids in the stomach. Relax after eating your meals. However, avoid lying down. Go for the relaxation techniques like meditation, yoga or deep breathing.

- **Avoid big meals at night or late night eating**

Make sure to have your last meal of the day at least 2-3 hours before bedtime. This will reduce your stomach acid while allowing the stomach to empty its contents partially before sleeping. Large meals can put pressure on the stomach. Therefore, try to have 5-6 small meals a day rather than three big meals. Also, avoid heavy meals late in the evening.

- **Remain upright after eating**

Staying upright after meals reduces the risk of the stomach acid flowing back into the esophagus. Also, avoid bending over or straining to lift heavy objects after eating meals.

- **Quit Smoking**

Smoking can worsen the symptoms of heartburn. It not only irritates the GI tract, but also relaxes the muscles in the esophagus that play a role in keeping stomach acid in its place and preventing its regurgitation.

- **Reduce your intake of caffeine**

It has been found that many people complain of acid reflux after drinking coffee. Most patients report having obtained substantial relief after reducing their intake of coffee. Hence, you are advised to limit your leisurely cup of coffee for weekend breakfast in order to avoid the symptoms of acid reflux.

- **Wait before Exercise**

Exercise and regular workouts are the best ways to deal with any health issue. However, when you are suffering from acid reflux or heartburn, it is important to make sure you maintain a gap of at least half an hour between the time you eat a meal and when you exercise.

- **Sleep Position**

When you lie down flat in your bed, the throat and stomach stay at the same level. This makes it easier for the acid to flow back into the esophagus, thus leading to heartburn. It is, therefore, suggested to elevate your upper body while sleeping. This can be done in two ways:

Put the head-side of the bed on 5 to 6 inch blocks, or Try to sleep on a wedge-shaped pillow. The pillow should be at least 6 to 8 inches thick on one side. However, avoid substituting the wedge pillow with regular pillows because they just raise the head and not the entire upper body.

If you don't find that these lifestyle changes help and are effective in reducing the symptoms of heartburn or acid reflux, then it is time to go see a doctor and start taking medication to solve the problem. Indications that will let you know it's time to consult a doctor might include symptoms like continuous and untreated eructations, difficulty in swallowing, vomiting due to heartburn and continued heartburn even after using antacids for as long as two weeks.

Conclusion

Thank you again for downloading this book!

I hope this book has enabled you to stop the symptoms of acid reflux or GERD and therefore improve your quality of life

The next step is to use the methods discussed in this book and make the necessary diet and life style changes that will enable you to rid yourself of the symptoms of acid reflux and GERD forever!

Part 2

What is acid reflux?

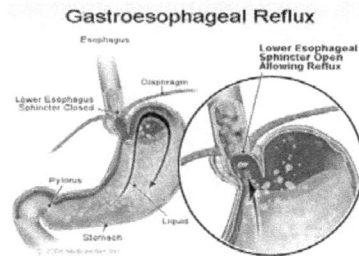

Gastroesophageal Reflux

Acid reflux, which is also known as gastroesophageal reflux disease (GERD), is a condition in which some of the liquid content of the stomach refluxes, regurgitates, or moves back up into the esophagus. Since this liquid may be acidic, it can damage and inflame the lining of the esophagus (a condition which is known as esophagitis. In a minority of patients suffering from acid refluxes, there are visible signs of inflammation. The regurgitated liquid that moves into the esophagus contains pepsin and acid contents that are produced by the stomach. Pepsin is an enzyme that initiates the digestion or breakdown of proteins in the stomach.

Apart from pepsin and acid, the refluxed liquid can also contain a little amount of bile that has backed-up from the duodenum into the stomach. The duodenum is the first segment of the small intestine that is attached to the stomach. The most harmful component of the refluxed liquid is known to be the acid present in it.

Although bile and pepsin can also injure the esophagus, their role in the inflammation and damage of esophageal is not as visible as that of acid.

GERD is known to be a chronic condition because it usually is life-long once it begins. Once this leads to esophagitis (damage to the lining or coating of the esophagus), another chronic condition is set to develop. Esophagitis is a chronic condition because its treatment never stops. Once the condition is healed with a particular treatment, and the treatment is stopped, the condition or injury will return in a few months in most patients. This simply means that once you initiate the treatment for GERD, you will have to continue the treatment indefinitely. However, some people suffering from acid reflux and with intermittent symptoms (with no signs of esophagitis) can be treated intermittently (that is only during symptomatic periods).

We all experience acid reflux; this means that the reflux of the liquid contents from the stomach into the esophagus occurs in almost every normal individual. According to a study, it was found that reflux occurs regularly in normal persons as in patients suffering from GERD. However, in patients with GERD, the refluxed liquid has more acid content, and the content remains in the esophagus longer. Also, the liquid refluxes in patients with GERD move to a higher level in their esophagus than normal individuals.

As we all know, the body has ways of protecting itself from the acid and the harmful effects of reflux when it occurs. For example, most acid refluxes occur during the day, and when we are standing in most cases when we are upright. The body is doing this because when we are in the upright position, the refluxed liquid can flow back into the stomach more rapidly due to the effect of gravity. Also, acid reflux occurs mostly when people are awake; this is because we repeatedly swallow, whether there is acid reflux or not.

If there is reflux, each swallow will return the refluxed liquid into the stomach before it causes any inflammation or danger. Lastly, the salivary glands that are present in our mouths produce saliva. This saliva contains bicarbonate. Once we swallow when we are awake, the bicarbonate-containing saliva goes down through the esophagus. While on the way, the bicarbonate neutralizes the little amount of acid that is present in the esophagus after swallowing, and gravity has removed most of the acidic reflux liquid.

Although saliva, swallowing, and gravity are the three main protective mechanisms that the body is using to protect the esophagus, they are only effective when we are in the upright position or when we are fully awake. When we are sleeping at night, swallowing stops, gravity does not affect, and the rate at which the body is secreting saliva is reduced. This simply means that if anyone of us is to experience acid reflux, it will start when sleeping. When acid reflux occurs at night, there is a higher probability that there will be remains of acid in the esophagus longer than expected. This will lead to a more significant injury or damage to the esophagus.

Certain conditions will make a person susceptible to GERD. Also, we have different conditions that may lead to having higher degrees of acid reflux. For example, there may be a severe acid reflux condition during pregnancy. What is expected to cause this problem is the elevated hormone levels that occur during pregnancy. This will cause reflux because it causes a reduction in the pressure in the lower esophageal sphincter.

This is in addition to the increase in pressure that is caused by the growing fetus in the abdomen. Both of these conditions are known to boost the presence of reflux in pregnant women. Another example occurs in patients with diseases that reduce the strength of their esophageal muscles, such as mixed connective tissue diseases or scleroderma. These people are more prone to the development of acid reflux disease.

GERD in infants

Many babies are suffering from GERD, and about two-thirds of 4-month-old babies are showing the symptoms of GERD. In addition to this, up to 10 percent of 1-year-old babies are also showing signs of acid reflux. Normally, it is good for babies to vomit and spit-up food sometimes. However, once your baby is vomiting or spitting up food frequently, there is a probability that they have acid reflux. Other potential symptoms and signs of GERD in infants include difficulty sleeping, weight loss or poor growth, trouble swallowing, wet burps or hiccups, irritability during or after feeding, and refusal to eat. Recurring cough or pneumonia, arching of their back during or after eating or feeding them and gagging or choking.

Many of these signs and symptoms are also found in infants that have tongue-tie. This is a condition that can make it hard for them to shout when crying or eating. You need to make an appointment with your doctor once you suspect anything strange with your child, especially when you suspect that he or she may have a health condition. When you visit your doctor, you will also learn more from them, like how to recognize GERD in infants.

Risk factors for GERD

Certain conditions can boost your chances of developing acid reflux. Some of these conditions include hiatal hernia, pregnancy, obesity, and connective tissue disorders. Some lifestyle behaviors that can also increase the rate at which you suffer from acid reflux include eating large meals, smoking, going to sleep or lying down shortly after eating, and eating certain kinds of foods, such as spicy foods or deep-fried. Others include drinking certain types of beverages like coffee, soda, or alcohol, and using NSAIDs (nonsteroidal anti-inflammatory drugs) such as ibuprofen or aspirin. If you have any of the above risk factors, you need to take bold steps to modify them in a way to manage or prevent acid reflux.

Anxiety and GERD

According to data released by researchTrusted Source in 2015, anxiety might make some or all of the symptoms of acid reflux to get worse. If you suspect that fearing or having anxiety is making your acid reflux symptoms worse, you must consider booking an appointment with your doctor. Your doctor will provide a solution and strategies to relieve it. Some of the things you need to do to reduce anxiety are as follows:

• adjust your exercise routine, sleep habits, or other lifestyle behaviors

• practice relaxation techniques, like deep breathing exercises or meditation

• limit your exposure to people, experiences, and places that you think are making you feel anxious

You may be referred to a mental health specialist for evaluation, diagnosis, and treatment if he suspects that you have an anxiety disorder. Some of the treatments that you can use for anxiety disorder might include therapy talk, medication, or a combination of both.

Pregnancy and GERD

There is a higher probability of experiencing acid reflux in people who are pregnant. Having pregnant can increase your chances of having higher and more severe acid reflux symptoms. If you are suffering from acid reflux or GERD before you get pregnant, there is a higher probability of you having worse symptoms of the condition. What is responsible for the worsening of the symptoms is the changes in your hormones during pregnancy.

This changes will lead to having the muscles in your esophagus to relax more frequently; this will thereby cause easy flowing of stomach liquid into the esophagus. In addition to this, a growing fetus in your stomach can lead to an increase in the pressure on your stomach. All these can lead to an increase in the rate at which stomach acid will be entering your esophagus.

Asthma and GERD

According to recent research, it has been shown that more than 75 percent of people who are suffering from asthma also experience acid reflux or GERD. There have been several studies on the relationship between asthma and acid reflux or GERD; all these studies will help to understand the relationship and the solution or treatment. The symptoms of acid reflux might be worse than the symptoms of asthma. However, the medications you can use for asthma can raise your risk of experiencing acid reflux. It is important to manage your conditions if you have asthma and GERD. You need to contact your doctor for more information on how to manage your condition because it is not easy to manage.

Irritable Bowel Syndrome (IBS) and GERD

Irritable bowel syndrome (also known as IBS) is a condition that mainly affects the large intestine. Some of the symptoms of this condition include bloating, diarrhea, constipation, and abdominal pain. People with irritable bowel syndrome are known to suffer more GERD-related symptoms than the general population; this is according to reviewTrusted Source. You need to make an appointment with a doctor if you have symptoms of both GERD and irritable bowel syndrome. Your doctor might recommend that you change your medications, diet, or other treatments.

Drinking alcohol and GERD

Some specific foods and drinks will worsen your symptoms when you are among those suffering from acid reflux. Some of the diets that may trigger your acid reflux symptoms include alcoholic beverages. You might have to drink alcohol in moderation, depending on your specific triggers. For some people, even having a taste of alcohol can trigger their symptoms of acid reflux.

If alcohol is combined with fruit juices or other mixers, the combination might also trigger symptoms. There are different ways you can manage this combination to prevent this from triggering GERD symptoms. Contact your doctor for more information on how to manage yourself. If you must drink alcohol, there are different ways you can manage yourself, but you shouldn't drink it. Contact your doctor and let him help you with a better solution.

Causes of Acid Reflux

*A*lthough many people may think that there is nothing much associated with the production of acid reflux in the esophagus from the lungs, this is not true as there are many causes of acid reflux. The cause of GERD is complex. In this case, acid reflux involves multiple causes. Different causes of acid reflux usually affect different people in different ways or even in the same person in different ways and at different times. While a small number of people suffering from acid reflux may abnormally produce large amounts of acid, this is not very common among the people. It is also not a contributing factor in most people suffering from acid reflux.

The main factors that contribute to GERD include Hiatal hernias, slow or extended emptying of the stomach, lower esophageal sphincter abnormalities, and abnormal esophageal contractions. All these are what make GERD happen and get worse with time. You need to know more about these factors to get to know about acid reflux or GERD.

Hiatal hernia

Although their way of contribution is not very clear, Hiatal hernias are known to contribute to reflux. While the majority of people suffering from reflux have Hiatal hernias, many of them do not have. This simply shows that it is not compulsory to have a hiatal hernia when you are suffering from GERD. Also, suffering from GERD does not mean that you must have a Hiatal hernia. In contrast, many people have Hiatal hernias, and they are not suffering from GERD. There is no certain reason why this leads to the development of hiatal hernia.

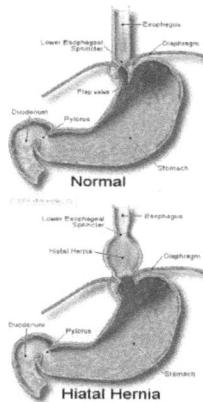

Normal

Hiatal Hernia

Typically, the lower esophageal sphincter is located precisely at the same level, where the esophagus goes through the chest into the abdomen through a small passage in the diaphragm. If you don't know, the diaphragm is a muscular, horizontal partition that is separating the abdomen from the chest. When someone is suffering from hiatal hernia, a small part of the upper stomach, which is linked with the esophagus, goes up into the chest through the diaphragm. This will result in having a small part of the lower esophageal sphincter and the stomach to come to lie in the chest. With this, the lower esophageal sphincter will no longer be at the level of the diaphragm again.

From the picture of hiatal hernia, the diaphragm that surrounds the lower esophageal sphincter is the most crucial part that helps in preventing reflux from the stomach. This simply means that in people without Hiatal hernias, there is a continuous contraction of the diaphragm that surrounds the esophagus, but it relaxes with swallows just like the lower esophageal sphincter. You should also note that the effects of the diaphragm and the lower esophageal sphincter occur at the same point in people with GERD but without Hiatal hernias.

Therefore, the barrier to acid reflux is the same as the pressures that are generated by both the lower esophageal sphincter and the diaphragm. The lower esophageal sphincter and the diaphragm will continue to exert their barrier effect and pressures when the lower esophageal sphincter moves into the chest in people with hiatal hernia, although this is now occurring at different locations.

Consequently, the compressions are no longer additive. Instead of this, a single high-pressure barricade to acid reflux is replaced by two barricades of lower pressure, and this makes reflux to occur more easily than before. So, the only way through which hiatal hernia can contribute to reflux is by decreasing the pressure barrier.

Lower esophageal sphincter

The working principle of the lower esophageal sphincter (LES) is possibly the most important mechanism or factor for preventing reflux. As we already know that the esophagus is a muscular tube that goes from the base of the throat, and it extends to the stomach; the lower esophageal sphincter is a specialized ring of muscle. This muscle is the muscle that surrounds the lower-most part of the esophagus (the part which joins the stomach).

However, there is an active muscle that made up the lower esophageal sphincter, and this muscle is always at rest. This means that this muscle is always contracting, and it closes off the passage that links the esophagus into the stomach. In other words, the closing of this passage helps to avoid or prevent reflux. However, when we are eating, the muscle at the lower esophageal sphincter relaxes for some seconds, thereby allowing saliva or food to go through into the stomach through the esophagus, and then it closes again.

With these actions of the lower esophageal sphincter, people with GERD are known to possess different abnormalities of the LES, and this is one of the reasons why they are having issues with reflux. Two of these abnormalities are involved in the function of the lower esophageal sphincter. The first is abnormal relaxations of the lower esophageal sphincter, which is called transient LES relaxations, and the second one is the abnormally weak contraction of the lower esophageal sphincter, which reduces the ability of it to prevent or get rid of reflux.

What makes them abnormal is that they do not allow and accompany swallows, and their inability to contract lasts for a long time (which can be up to several minutes). This inability allows easy reoccurrence of reflux easily. The temporary lower esophageal sphincter relaxations occur in people suffering from reflux most commonly after eating, that is when the stomach is expanded with food. Although temporary lower esophageal sphincter relaxations also occur in people who are not suffering from reflux, they are infrequent.

Laxity of the lower esophageal sphincter is the most recently-described abnormality in people suffering from reflux or GERD. In short, comparable distending pressures open the lower esophageal sphincter more in people with GERD than in people without GERD. This will allow smooth opening of the lower esophageal sphincter when the lower esophageal sphincter is open and greater backward flow of acid into the esophagus.

Esophageal contractions

As we already know that swallows are essential when it comes to the elimination of acid in the esophagus. There is a ring-like wave of contraction in the muscles of the esophagus when swallowing, and this narrows the inner cavity (lumen) of the esophagus. This contraction is also known as peristalsis, and it begins in the upper esophagus immediately after swallowing, and it extends down to the lower esophagus. This contraction pushes saliva, food, and anything that you put into your stomach that passes through the esophagus into the stomach.

Now, when there is a defection in the wave of contraction, there will be an inability of the refluxed acid to be pushed back into the stomach. In people who are suffering from acid reflux, there has been the presence of several abnormalities of contraction. For instance, the waves of contraction may die out before they extend or travel to the stomach, or the waves of contraction may not start immediately after each swallow. In addition to this, the pressure that is generated by the contractions may not be too strong to push back the refluxed acid into the stomach.

Abnormalities of contraction like these that reduce the pushing of the refluxed acid from the esophagus to the stomach are seen regularly in patients with GERD. These abnormalities are found most frequently in people who are suffering from acid reflux. The time when the effects of the abnormal esophageal contractions are expected to be worse is at night when there is no gravity. This is because gravity helps to return refluxed acid into the stomach. Please, also note that people who are smoking have an increased reduction in the ability to clear the acid from the esophagus. Smoke affects this, and the effect goes on to at least six hours after smoking the last cigarette.

Emptying of the stomach

Most acid refluxes that occur during the day occur after meals. This acid reflux occurs possibly due to the temporary lower esophageal sphincter LES relaxations. These relaxations are caused mainly by the distention of the stomach with food. A smaller number of people who are suffering from GERD have been known to have abnormal emptying of their stomachs after a meal. This is called gastroparesis. This abnormal emptying is very slow, and it prolongs the distention of the stomach after meals with food, and this increases the chance of getting acid reflux.

This shows that reflux is more expected to occur during the prolonged emptying of the stomach. We have several medications that are associated with impaired gastric emptying. Some of these medications include calcium channel blockers (CCBs), tricyclic antidepressants, dopamine agonists, narcotics, clonidine, nicotine, lithium (Eskalith, Lithobid), and progesterone.

As a GERD patient, if you are prescribed any of these drugs, you should not stop taking these drugs that are prescribed to you. This must continue until the prescribing doctor can diagnose you and tell you the current state of your GERD. This way, he or she will describe another drug for you or give you other drugs to use.

Symptoms of uncomplicated Acid Reflux?

There are several symptoms of uncomplicated GERD, but below are the three primary symptoms. These include nausea, regurgitation, and heartburn (which is sometimes known as chest pain). Other symptoms of GERD comes with the complications of GERD. This way, they will be discussed in line with the complications.

Nausea
Nausea is not very common in GERD. However, it has been seen in many patients who have severe or frequent nausea, which usually results in vomiting. One of the first conditions to be considered in people who are suffering from unexplained nausea or vomiting is GERD. However, there is no clear explanation as to why some patients with GERD develop mainly nausea, and others develop mainly heartburn. This may depend on the patient, and it may not be general. This way, you will have to be diagnosed first before treatment concerning your type of acid reflux symptoms to be treated.

Regurgitation
Regurgitation is a situation whereby the refluxed liquid appeared in the mouth. In many patients with GERD, only a small amount of the refluxed liquid will reach the esophagus while the remaining refluxed liquid remains in the lower part of the esophagus. Sometimes in many patients suffering from GERD, larger amounts of refluxed liquid which do contain food particles reach the upper esophagus.

The upper esophageal sphincter (UES) is located very close to the mouth at the upper end of the esophagus. The upper esophageal sphincter, UES is a circular ring of muscle which is very similar in look and actions to the lower esophageal sphincter, LES. This simply means that the action of the upper esophageal sphincter helps to prevent the presence of the refluxed liquid in the throat.

When little quantity of the refluxed liquid (with or without the food content) get past the upper esophageal sphincter and enter the throat of the patient, there may be the taste of acid in the mouth. If the upper esophageal sphincter allows larger quantities of the refluxed liquid into their mouth, such patients may find the liquid or food full in their mouths. With this, prolonged or frequent regurgitation can lead to having teeth that are induced with acid erosions.

Heartburn
Nerve fibers that are present in the esophagus are stimulated when the acid refluxes into the esophagus from the stomach in people suffering from GERD. The stimulation of the nerve is what commonly results in heartburn. The heartburn is one of the characteristics of GERD. If you don't know, heartburn is known as the burning pain that is located in the middle of the chest. This pain of heartburn may extend up into the neck when it starts high in the abdomen. In some other GERD patients, the pain may be pressure-like or very sharp rather than burning. Pain like this can mimic

heart pain (which is also known as angina). The pain may extend to the back in many other patients.

However, since acid reflux always happens after meals, heartburn also occurs after meals. However, since acid reflux occurs more at night when there is no gravity, heartburn is also common when these people lie down or when they are sleeping. This is because the acid return more slowly into the stomach due to lack of gravity. Many people suffering from acid reflux are awakened from their sleep when the pain of heartburn occur to them.

Episodes of heartburn seem to happen periodically. This statement means that the episodes of heartburn occur more frequently or severely for weeks or months. On the other hand, the pain becomes less severe or frequent or even fade away for several weeks or months. This periodic change in the symptoms gives room for intermittent treatment in people with GERD and with the absent of esophagitis. However, heartburn is a life-long problem that will always return after weeks or months of absence.

Complications of Acid Reflux

There are many complications of acid reflux, and below are some of them.

Ulcers

There are a lot of cells that are lining the esophagus, and these cells are damaged by the liquid that is refluxed from the stomach into the esophagus. When this happens, the body will react to the damage the same way it reacts to damages that occur with inflammation (this inflammation is also known as esophagitis). This inflammation is a process that involves the neutralization of the damaging agent, cleaning the place of harmful materials and begin the process of healing as soon as possible. If this damage extends into the esophagus, there will be the formation of an ulcer. In simple meaning, an ulcer is damage that is caused in the lining of the esophagus in the area of inflammation.

When ulcer occurs, the additional inflammation that comes with it may erode into the blood vessels around the esophagus, thereby leading to the bleeding into the esophagus. This is a severe issue, and when the bleeding is severe, there may be the need for surgical treatment, blood transfusions, or an endoscopic procedure. The endoscopic procedure is a procedure whereby a tube is passed into the esophagus through the mouth to visualize the bleeding site and to stop the bleeding. These are the only solutions available for ulcers in the esophagus.

Strictures

What makes ulcers of the esophagus heal is the formation of scars or otherwise known as fibrosis. The scar tissue will shrink over time, and it will narrow the inner cavity or the lumen of the esophagus. The narrowing of the inner cavity of the esophagus is what is called a stricture. The stricture may lead to painful swallowing of food once the narrowing becomes severe enough. The severity occurs when the scar has restricted the esophageal lumen or inner cavity to a diameter which is less than one centimeter. This condition may lead to the endoscopic or surgical removal of the food that got stuck. To prevent this from happening, the scars may be reduced, or the narrowing must be widened (or stretched). In addition to this and to prevent the future occurrence of the stricture, the doctor must find a better way to prevent reflux.

Barrett's esophagus

Long term, severe, or prolonged GERD causes variations in the cells that are lining the esophagus in some people suffering from acid reflux. These cells are known to be pre-cancerous, and they may soon become cancerous. The condition we just described is known as Barrett's esophagus, and it is usually known to be present among up to 10% of patients suffering from GERD. There is a rapid increase in the type of esophageal cancer that is linked with Barrett's esophagus (it is also known as adenocarcinoma). While many people suffering from acid reflux develop Barrett's esophagus, this condition cannot be explained yet, and most patients with GERD do not develop Barrett's esophagus.

To confirm the presence of Barrett's esophagus, doctors confirm this condition visually during the time of endoscopy, and this condition is confirmed with the use of microscopic examination of the cells lining the esophagus. After the confirmation, the patient that develop Barrett's esophagus can experience periodic surveillance endoscopies with biopsies. Even though there is no reasonable agreement to which these people will require surveillance. The main reason why they are putting patients under surveillance is to notice the progression from the current stage (pre-cancerous stage) to the more cancerous stage so that there will be the initiation of the cancer treatment. This will help to prevent or reduce the maximum growth of cancer.

However, it is also better that people suffering from Barrett's esophagus must receive maximum treatment for acid reflux. This type of treatment will help prevent further damage or harm to the esophagus. Current studies are going on to assist in the removal of the abnormal lining cells in the esophagus. They are now using different endoscopic, non-surgical techniques to get rid of the cells. Although these techniques are the best because they do not require surgery for the removal, they come with complications. However, the long-term effectiveness of this type of treatment is yet to be determined. The best option is for the removal of the esophagus is always the use of surgery.

Cough and asthma

There are many nerves present in the lower part of the esophagus, and the refluxed acid stimulates many of these nerves. The stimulation of these nerves results in pain (usually as a result of heartburn). Other stimulated nerves in the esophagus do not produce pain. They will, instead, stimulate other nerves that will provoke coughing. This simply means that there may be coughing in people suffering from acid reflux, which may not even get to the throat.

On the other hand, but similarly, reflux into the lower part of the esophagus can stimulate the nerves of the esophagus that connects to the lungs. This will also stimulate nerves that lead to the lungs. These stimulated nerves in the lungs can lead to the narrowing of the smaller breathing tubes. This will then result in an attack of asthma.

Although acid reflux may cause cough in most patients, it is not a common cause of mysterious coughing. Also, acid reflux may cause asthma, and it may increase asthmatic attacks in people who already have asthma. Although asthma and chronic cough are common disorders, no evidence shows that they are caused or aggravated by acid reflux.

Inflammation of the larynx and throat
The reflux liquid can enter the voice box (larynx) or even the throat (pharynx) when it moves past the upper esophageal sphincter. Once this happens, it may lead to inflammation that can lead to hoarseness and a sore throat. Just like coughing and asthma, we cannot show that acid reflux is one of the factors responsible for the inflammation of the larynx and the throat.

Infection and inflammation of the lungs

When liquid from the stomach refluxed, and it passes through the throat (pharynx) into the voice box (larynx), it can enter the lungs (aspiration). When this occurs in the lungs (aspiration), the refluxed liquid can lead to coughing and choking. However, aspiration can also occur without the production of any of these symptoms. Aspiration may lead to infection or inflammation of the lungs with or without these symptoms, and this can and result in pneumonia.

Pneumonia that is caused by a situation like this is a serious one, and it requires immediate treatment. There may be pulmonary fibrosis (progressive scarring of the lungs) when there is aspiration without the presence of symptoms, and this can only be seen on chest X-rays. The only time that aspiration occurs most is at night when there is no active processes or mechanism that will protect you against reflux. This is also the time that there is no active coughing reflex that will protect the lungs.

Fluid in the middle ears and sinuses

There is always communication that is going on between the throat and the nasal passages. There are adenoids (two patches of lymph tissue) at the upper part of the throat, and it joins the nasal passages in small children. The passages from the Eustachian tubes (the tubes from the middle ears) and the sinuses open into the rear part of the nasal passages very close to the adenoids. However, the liquid that refluxed from the stomach can enter the upper throat to aggravate the adenoids and cause them to enlarge or swell.

The swollen adenoids can then obstruct the passages from the Eustachian tubes and the sinuses. When the middle ears and the sinuses are blocked from the nasal passages due to the swelling of the adenoids, there will be an accumulation of fluids within them. The accumulation of fluid in them can lead to pain and discomfort in the ears and the sinuses. However, this condition is not seen in adults but children because adenoids are noticeable in young children. So, when your children are complaining of pains in their ears, you should take them to the hospital for diagnosis and treatment before something else starts developing in them.

How is acid reflux diagnosed and evaluated?

When it comes to diagnosing and evaluating patients with GERD, there are different tests, procedures, and evaluations of symptoms (like heartburn) to be used.

- **Symptoms and procedures to diagnose acid reflux.**

- **Symptoms and response to treatment (otherwise called therapeutic trial).**

Heartburn is the usual way that they are describing acid reflux. Heartburn is usually described as a sub-sternal (occurring under the middle of the chest) pain or burning that occurs after eating due to reflux, and it often worsens when lying down. The best method of treatment that physicians are using is by prescribing patients with medications that will hinder or reduce the production of the acid by the stomach. If the use of the medication can suppress the pain to a large extent, it means that the physician will confirm the diagnosis of GERD. This type of approach in diagnosing a type of condition based on the response of the body to the treatment of symptoms is commonly called a therapeutic trial.

However, since this is a trial, there are issues with this approach. For example, people who are suffering from conditions that can mimic acid reflux, such as gastric (stomach) or duodenal ulcers, can respond to such treatment. If the physician thereby confirms the condition to be acid reflux, he or she might have missed the treatment of ulcer disease. What usually causes such an ulcer is a type of infection called nonsteroidal anti-inflammatory drugs, Helicobacter pylori (H. pylori), or NSAIDs (such as ibuprofen). All of these can cause ulcer disease, and they would be treated differently from acid reflux.

However, when it comes to any treatment, there will be up to 20% placebo effect. This means that 20% of patients will respond to an inactive (placebo) pill or any form of treatment. On the other hand, this means that up to 20% of the people who are experiencing symptoms from other problems apart from acid reflux will have to respond to the treatment and thus have a reduced symptom effect. This means that after the therapeutic trial, these people will be subjected to the treatment of acid reflux when they do not have acid reflux. This simply means that the cause of their symptoms and their problems will not be pursued and be treated.

Endoscopy

One common way of diagnosing acid reflux is through the use of esophageal-gastro-duodenoscopy or EGD (it is also known as upper gastrointestinal endoscopy). Upper gastrointestinal endoscopy is a procedure through which a tube that contains an optical system that will be used for visualization is swallowed or inserted into the esophagus of the patient. As the tube is going down through the gastrointestinal tract, the walls or lining of the esophagus, the stomach, and the duodenum can all be examined.

Most patients suffering from acid reflux have esophagi that look normal. This simply means that endoscopy will not be the best solution in the diagnosis of GERD in most patients. On the other hand, the lining of the esophagus of these patients will appear inflamed (a condition known as esophagitis). Moreover, if ulcers (deeper breaks or damages in the lining) or erosions (superficial breaks or damages in the esophageal lining) are seen, you can confirm the presence of acid reflux confidently.

The use of endoscopy will also display different complications of acid reflux, especially Barrett's esophagus, strictures, and ulcers. Biopsies also may be obtained. Lastly, other common problems that may be associated with acid reflux can be diagnosed with upper gastrointestinal endoscopy. Some of these include inflammation, ulcers, or cancers of the duodenum or stomach.

Biopsies

The use of the endoscope for the result of the biopsies of the esophagus are not known to be very useful for diagnosing acid reflux. However, they are useful for the diagnosis of cancers or many other causes of esophageal inflammation and infections apart from acid reflux. Moreover, biopsies are only very useful for diagnosing the cellular variations of Barrett's esophagus.

According to recent research, it has been shown that people who are suffering from acid reflux whose esophagi appear normal will show widening and enlargement of the spaces among the lining cells; this is possibly an indication of damage in the cells. Although we cannot conclude now that seeing enlargement or widening between the cells confirms the presence of acid reflux, with this, another test will be carried out to confirm the presence of acid reflux or GERD.

X-rays

X-rays of the esophagus (which is also known as esophageal) used to be the only way of diagnosing GERD or acid reflux before the introduction of endoscopy. People suffering from acid reflux will have to swallow barium (which is a contrast material), and they will have to take the X-ray of the barium-filled esophagus. Although they were using it like that, esophageal has one main problem; the problem is that it is insensitive to the presence of acid reflux.

This simply means that it is a test that is failed to detect any failing signs of acid reflux in many patients. This is because the patients who are suffering from acid reflux have little or no damage caused to the lining of their esophagus. The use of X-rays will be able to show the infrequent complications of acid reflux, such as strictures and ulcers. Now, they have abandoned the use of X-rays for the diagnosing of acid reflux because of their inability to show positive results, although they are still using X-rays along with endoscopy for the evaluation of complications.

Examination of the larynx and throat

When acid reflux affects the larynx and the throat and leads to the symptoms of hoarseness, cough, or sore throat, the affected person can pay a visit to a nose, ear, and throat (ENT) specialist. This is because this specialist will be able to find signs of inflammation or irritation of the larynx or throat. Although this type of inflammation may be caused by the diseases of the larynx or throat, sometimes acid reflux may be the main cause. Accordingly, these specialists will have to try the use of acid-suppressing treatment on the patient to confirm the diagnosis of acid reflux. The result of this will help to confirm the presence of GERD and to start every possible form of treatment on the patient.

Acid Reflux (GERD) Tests

Esophageal acid testing

This is one of the best acid reflux tests that are available nowadays. Esophageal acid testing is known to be a "gold standard" for diagnosing acid reflux (GERD). As we already know, the reflux of acid from the stomach is a common condition in the general population. However, people suffering from acid reflux and the complications or symptoms of acid reflux have more reflux of acid from their stomach more than normal individuals who do not have the complications or symptoms of GERD. Moreover, we can distinguish patients with GERD from normal individuals by the amount of acid that is present in their esophagus.

To get the amount of time that the acid is left in the esophagus is determined by a test that is known as a 24-hour esophageal pH test. pH is known generally as a mathematical way of determining and expressing the amount of acidity. To carry out this test, a catheter (which is a small tube) is passed through the nose and allow to rest in the esophagus. They will place a sensor that senses acid at the tip of the catheter that is inside the esophagus.

The other part of the catheter that comes out from the nose is wrapped back over the ear and passed down over to the waist. This end is attached to a recorder at the waist. The recorder at the other end will have to record the episode of reflux when there is a reflux of acid from the stomach into the esophagus, and the sensor senses its presence. After recording the episodes for some time (say about 20 to 24 hours), the catheter will be removed, and they will analyze the record of reflux that was shown by the recorder.

There are a lot of issues associated with the use of pH testing for diagnosing acid reflux or GERD. Although it is possible to separate patients with GERD from normal individuals fairly well when they use a pH test, the separation is not perfect. This simply means that some people who are suffering from GERD will have the normal amount, and the same flow of acid reflux like a normal person and people without GERD may have abnormal or irregular amounts of acid reflux.

Therefore, to test for the presence of GERD, there is a need for something more than a pH test for confirmation. Examples of what can be used for this test are the presence of complications of GERD, response to treatment, or typical symptoms that the person is showing. In another way, physicians may confidently diagnose GERD when episodes of heartburn move with acid reflux, as shown by the result of acid testing.

The use of pH testing is now more popular for the management of GERD than just for the diagnosing of GERD. For instance, the use of pH testing is now being used for the determination of the reason why a pertinent with GERD symptoms do not show positive results to treatment. This is because up to 20 % of the patients with GERD symptoms will not respond positively, and their symptoms will not improve, no matter the treatment they give them for their GERD. The inability of these people to respond to treatment could be because of the type of treatment they are receiving or ineffective treatment. This means that the person is not successfully diagnosed, and the medication is not suppressing the production of acid in the stomach adequately. In other words, this is not reducing acid reflux.

On the other hand, we can explain the lack of response by an incorrect or wrong diagnosis of GERD. In either of these situations, we can make use of a pH test; it will be beneficial. If the testing shows considerable reflux of acid while they are still using medication, then the treatment will need to be changed because that treatment is ineffective for the person. However, if the pH testing shows good acid suppression with reduced reflux of acid, there is likely to be a wrong diagnosis of GERD, and they need to look out for other causes for the symptoms. This will help to get a better treatment for the person.

We can use pH testing to determine the main cause of symptoms (usually heartburn) and whether reflux is the real cause. The best way to make this evaluation is by recording patient reading whenever they have symptoms while they are still doing the 24-hour pH testing. However, when they are still analyzing the test, they can determine whether acid reflux is occurring at the time of the symptoms or not. If there is a presence of reflux during the time the symptoms show, then the main cause of the symptoms is likely to be reflux. However, if there is no reflux when the patient shows the symptoms, then there is no assurance that the reflux is the main cause of the symptoms.

Lastly, they are now using pH testing to evaluate patients before surgical or endoscopic treatment for GERD. As we already know that there is always a placebo effect. This effect shows that some 20% of patients will show improvement in their symptoms when treated even though they do not have GERD. Before surgical or endoscopic treatment, it is better to identify and sort out these patients because they may not benefit from the treatments, and the treatment of them will be a waste. To identify and remove these patients, you can use pH study because they will have normal acid reflux in their esophagus.

There is now a newer method that makes use of a prolonged measurement (up to 48 hours). This measurement means that there will be a prolonged exposure of the acid in the esophagus for 48 hours. This method will make use of a small, wireless capsule. This capsule will be attached to the esophagus a little above the lower esophageal sphincter. To do this, the capsule will be attached to a tube and inserted through either the nose or the mouth to the lower esophagus.

The tube will be removed after attaching the capsule to the esophagus. The capsule will then be measuring the acid refluxing into the esophagus for 48 hours, and the information will be transferred into a receiver that is worn around the waist of the patient. The information recorded by the receiver will then be downloaded into a computer after 48 hours and then analyzed. After 3-5 days, the capsule will fall off the esophagus of the patient and will pass out from the anus in the stool. However, the capsule cannot be reused.

From the two methods, the capsule method has an advantage over the standard pH testing. This is because there is no anxiety over the passage and use of a catheter that passes through the nose and throat.

Moreover, patients look normal with the capsule because there is no catheter protruding from their mouths or noses. Once there is no tube passing through their mouths, they can go about their daily activities like going to work without having a feeling of self-conscious.

The use of the capsule is better because it records large data and for a more extended period (48 versus 24 hours) than the catheter. This gives more data on symptoms and acid reflux. With the additional information that it provides, physicians prefer the use of capsules than the use of a catheter.

Capsule pH testing is expensive. However, the capsules fall off prematurely sometimes, and they do not get attached to the esophagus easily. The receiver may not receive any signal from the capsule for some periods, and there may be a loss of information about the reflux of acid.

There is also a pain in swallowing after the attachment of the capsule; when this happens, the capsule may have to be removed endoscopically. Although the use of the capsule has its problems, it is a new technology that offers a solution to different problems concerning the diagnosing of GERD.

Esophageal motility testing

This type of testing is essential in the diagnosing of GERD. The esophageal motility testing is used to determine how perfectly the esophagus muscles are working. This will let us know the extent to which the wall of the esophagus is damaged. To carry out the motility testing, they will have to pass a thin tube (catheter) through the nostril of the patient and pass down to the back of the throat, and this will go through to the esophagus. The part of the catheter that is passed into the esophagus, there is an attachment of sensors that sense pressure.

When the esophagus muscle contracts, the pressure will be generated in them, and the sensors attached to the catheter will detect this pressure. The other end of the catheter that comes out of the nostril is then attached to a recorder. This recorder records the pressure. When the test is on, the pressure will be at rest, and the lower esophageal sphincter will be in a relaxed state. The relaxation is then evaluated. After that, the patient will have to swallows sips of water for the evaluation of the contractions of the esophagus.

There are two important uses of esophageal motility testing when it comes to the evaluation of GERD. The first use is in the evaluation of symptoms that fail to respond to the treatment offered for GERD. This is made possible because the unusual function of the esophageal muscle may lead to something similar to the symptoms of GERD. The use of mobility testing can help to identify some of these irregularities for better diagnosis and evaluation of an esophageal motility condition.

On the other hand, the second use of esophageal motility testing is for the evaluation before endoscopic or surgical treatment for GERD. The main reason behind this is to identify GERD patients who have motility disorders that are affecting the esophageal muscle. This means that surgeons will have to look for a better surgery for patients with motility disorders.

Gastric emptying studies
These are the studies that are used to determine the rate at which foods are emptied from the stomach. As we have already known, up to 20 % of people suffering from GERD have a lower rate of emptying of their stomach, and a situation like this will be contributing to the reflux of acid from the stomach. To start the gastric emptying studies, the patient will have to take a meal that is denoted with a radioactive substance. They will have to place a sensor that looks like a Geiger counter over the stomach. This will be used to measure the rate at which the radioactive substance present in the food empties from the stomach.

Information that they get from this emptying study will be used by the physicians to help patients manage their GERD. For example, if someone who is suffering from GERD is showing symptoms even after treatment with the usual medications, physicians will have to prescribe other medications that will increase the rate at which meals will be emptied from the stomach. On the other hand, they can do a surgical procedure in conjunction with GERD surgery to create a rapid way to empty the stomach. There is still a debate going on whether the finding of a way to reduce gastric emptying will help to boost the rate at which surgical treatment will help improve GERD.

Symptoms of vomiting, regurgitation, and nausea may be due either to GERD or an abnormal gastric emptying. To differentiate a patient whose symptoms are due to abnormal emptying of the stomach, the use of an evaluation of gastric emptying will be helpful.

Acid perfusion test

Bernstein or the acid perfusion test is a test used for determining if a chest pain suffered by a patient is caused by acid reflux. To perform the acid perfusion test, you will have to pass a thin tube through one nostril. The tube will go into the middle of the esophagus down the back of the throat. A dilute, physiologic salt solution (which is similar to the fluid that bathes the cells of the body) and acid solution are alternately perfused (poured) through the catheter and into the esophagus. When this is done, the patient will not know the type of solution that is being infused into their body. If the perfusion or pouring of the salt solution produces no pain and the pouring of the acid provokes the usual pain of the patient, the pain of the patient is likely to be caused by acid reflux.

However, the acid perfusion test is rarely used. The better test that is used for correlating acid reflux and pain is a pH capsule study or a 24-hour esophageal pH during which the patient's readings are taken at the time they are having pain. They will be able to see if there is an episode of acid reflux from the pH recorder. This is very important, especially if they need the recording at the time of the pain.

It offers the best way of deciding whether acid reflux is causing pain for the patient. However, if this does not go well for people who have infrequent pain, they can take a pH study every two to three days. In both cases, you can perform an acid perfusion test.

How is acid reflux (GERD) treated?

Lifestyle changes are one of the simplest treatments for acid reflux, and it is a mixture of several changes inhabit. The most important one is related to eating. Let us look at some ways through which acid reflux can be treated.

Lifestyle changes and acid reflux (GERD) diet

As we have already discussed, reflux of acid from the stomach is more severe and distressing at night than in the day. This is because when you are lying down, there is no gravity acting on your food, and it will be easier for acid reflux to occur. This is easier because gravity is not acting against the reflux, unlike when you are standing in an upright position during the day. Also, there is bound to be the traveling of the refluxed liquid from the stomach into the esophagus, and it will stay there for a long time because of the lack of the effect of gravity.

There are different ways to overcome these problems. You can elevate these problems by raising the upper body in bed partially. You can do this elevation either by placing a foam rubber wedge and sleeping with the upper body on it or by placing some blocks under the feet of your bed (at the head of the bed). These tricks are used to raise the esophagus higher than the stomach and somewhat try to restore the effects of gravity. What is very important here is that the upper part of your body should be elevated. This is because elevating the head alone will not elevate the esophagus, and this may not restore the effects of gravity on the body.

What is very important is that every patient with GERD must raise the upper part of their body at night. Nevertheless, most patients with acid reflux only experience reflux during the day, and they will have little stress, problem, and pain at night when they make use of elevation; this will benefit them. There is no way we can know which patient will benefit the use of elevation at night unless they make use of acid testing, which will clearly demonstrate night reflux.

On the other hand, patients who have regurgitation, heartburn, or other symptoms of acid reflux or GERD at night are probably experiencing reflux of the liquid from the stomach at night. This simply means that they should elevate their upper body when sleeping for their problem to ease. Reflux also occurs less regularly when GERD patients lie down using their left side rather than their right sides.

GERD diet
Another thing that can be useful in the treatment of GERD is making several changes in your eating habits. Reflux is worse after eating foods. This could probably be because the stomach is full and distended with food with all its muscles in distended modes. Also, there are frequent relaxations of the lower esophageal sphincter, giving room for smooth flowing back of the stomach liquid content in the esophagus. Therefore, eating your meals in smaller portions than two or three larger

portions of meals is recommended for people who are suffering from GERD.

Also, it is recommended that these patients eat evening meals earlier, like three hours before going to bed. All these may reduce the rate at which acid reflux occurs at night for two reasons. One, when they eat smaller meals, there will be lesser distention of the stomach, which will prevent easy flowing of the stomach content. Two, eating a smaller meal earlier will cause the food to be digested and would have emptied from the stomach faster than larger meals. This will, therefore, result in having lesser reflux in patients with GERD at night when they are sleeping, and they will be able to sleep well.

Certain foods are known to promote reflux because they are very good at reducing the pressure in the LES (lower esophageal sphincter). Patients suffering from GERD must avoid taking these foods by all means. These foods include chocolate, alcohol, peppermint, and caffeinated drinks. These people should also reduce the number of fatty foods in their diets, and they should stop smoking totally; this is because fatty foods and smoking are also known to promote reflux and reduce the pressure in the lower esophageal sphincter.

In addition to this, people suffering from GERD may get to know other foods that trigger or aggravate their symptoms. They should watch out for foods that are spicy and other acid-containing foods like tomato juice, carbonated beverages, and citrus juices. Since these foods are also known to provoke symptoms, they should be avoided by all means too.

One innovative approach for the treatment of GERD is for the GERD patient to be chewing gum. This is very important because chewing gum is known to increase the rate of swallowing while it promotes the production of bicarbonate-containing saliva in the mouth. The saliva neutralizes the acid that is present in the esophagus after it is swallowed. In effect, chewing gum is one of the normal processes that produce more saliva and neutralize the acid in the esophagus, although there is no current clear evidence to show that chewing gum is very effective in the treatment of heartburn. However, you can try chewing gum after meals; after all, it costs you nothing to try.

Acid reflux (GERD) medications

Apart from changing your lifestyles, there are a lot of OTC (over-the-counter) - such as antacids and foam barriers - and prescription medications - such as histamine antagonists, proton pump inhibitors, and promotility drugs - available for the treatment of GERD.

Antacids for GERD
Currently, antacids continue to be the mainstay of treatment for acid reflux despite the production of many potent medications that can be used for the treatment. This is because antacids perform the function of neutralizing the acid that is produced in the stomach and thereby preventing acid from refluxing into the esophagus. Although they are very effective for the treatment, they have a very brief action. This is because they are emptied faster from the empty stomach (say in an hour or less than an hour). When they are no more in the stomach, they give room for the production of the acid again.

However, to make them work better for you, the best time to take them is approximately one hour after eating your meals. This is just the time before you start feeling the symptoms of reflux after eating. Since the food taken will take a while before it is emptied from the stomach, the antacid that you take after a meal will stay longer, and as long as the food is in your stomach and it is effective longer. Also, you should take the second dose of antacids just about two hours after a meal. This will give it the ability to replace the first dose during the emptying of the stomach. It will improve the acid-neutralizing ability within the stomach.

Antacids may be calcium, magnesium, or aluminum-based. Unlike other antacids, calcium-based antacids (which are usually calcium carbonate) promote the release of gastrin from the duodenum and stomach. Gastrin primary hormone that is in control of the stimulation of acid production by the stomach. This means that the secretion of acid will continue after the calcium carbonate has finished its direct acid-neutralizing effect on the hormone. The reproduction of the acid is due to the release of gastrin after the antacids have stopped working, and this will lead to an overproduction of acid, as we all know that this increased acid production is not good for people suffering from GERD.

However, the reproduction of acid is yet to be proven clinically to be essential to the body. This simply means that treating GERD with calcium carbonate has not been confirmed to be less safe or effective than treatment with those antacids that are not containing calcium carbonate. Theoretically, the phenomenon of acid rebound is harmful to the body and GERD.

In practice, therefore, it is not recommended for patients with GERD to continue using calcium-containing antacids such as Rolaids and Tums. Although, the use of these calcium carbonate-containing antacids occasionally is not believed to be dangerous. Apart from stopping the production of acid, calcium carbonate-containing antacids are very advantageous because they add calcium to the body, they are low-cost, and they are convenient to use as compared to liquids.

On the other hand, aluminum-containing antacids can cause constipation when they are used to stop the production of acid in the stomach, while magnesium-containing antacids can cause diarrhea to the patient. If the patient started having constipation or diarrhea, it might be compulsory to switch antacids. Alternatively, you can use antacids that contain both magnesium and aluminum.

Histamine antagonists
Although antacids are known to be very effective in stopping the production of acids and neutralizing it, they do so only for a short time in the stomach. For a continuous neutralization of acid all through the day, GERD patients will have to be using antacids frequently, at least every hour.

Histamine antagonist, specifically Tagamet (cimetidine), was the first medication produced for the convenient and effective treatment of acid-related diseases such as GERD. Histamine is a vital chemical in the body because it enhances the production of acid by the stomach. When produced, histamine is released within the wall of the stomach, and it is attached to the binders (receptors) on the acid-producing cells in the stomach; it will then stimulate the cells for acid production.

The work of the histamine antagonists, on the other hand, is to block the receptor for histamine, thereby preventing the acid-producing cells from being stimulated for the production of acid. (since the specific receptor that histamine antagonists blocked is the histamine type 2 receptor, histamine antagonists are known as H2 antagonists).

Since histamine is very important for the production of acid after meals, the best time to take H2 antagonists is 30 minutes before meals. This is because the H2 antagonists will be working at their peak levels in the stomach after a meal and stop the stomach from producing acid. This timing must not be missed for the medication to be effective. Patients with GERD can also use H2 antagonists before going to be to reduce or stop the production of acid when they are sleeping.

The best medication that is very good for the relieving of the symptoms of GERD (especially heartburn) is the H2 antagonists. On the other hand, they are not very effective for the healing of esophagitis (inflammation that may accompany GERD). H2 antagonists are primarily used for the treatment of heartburn in acid reflux, even though it is not associated with complications or inflammation like strictures, ulcers, or Barrett's esophagus.

There are four different H2 antagonists available for the treatment of GERD by prescription; these include nizatidine (Axid), ranitidine (Zantac), cimetidine (Tagamet), and famotidine, (Pepcid). Even though they are all available over-the-counter (OTC) without the need for the doctor's prescription, the dosages offered at OTC are lower than those prescribed by the physicians and doctors.

Proton pump inhibitors

Proton pump inhibitor (PPI) (also known as omeprazole - Prilosec) is another and the second type of drug that is produced specifically for the treatment of acid-related diseases such as acid reflux (GERD). A proton pump inhibitor helps to stop or block the production and secretion of acid by the acid-secreting cells into the stomach. Although both proton pump inhibitors and H2 antagonists work well, PPI has an advantage over the H2 antagonist.

The advantage of a proton pump inhibitor over an H2 antagonist is that the proton pump inhibitor shuts off acid production completely and maintains this for a longer period. Not only that proton pump inhibitor is good for relieving the patient from the symptom of heartburn, but it is also perfect for the protection of the esophagus from acid. This will help in the healing of the esophageal inflammation.

Proton pump inhibitors are used when H2 antagonists are not relieving the patient off the symptoms or when complications of acid reflux such as Barrett's esophagus, erosions or ulcers, or strictures exist. Five different proton pump inhibitors are approved for the treatment of acid reflux or GERD. These include esomeprazole (Nexium), and pantoprazole (Protonix), lansoprazole (Prevacid), rabeprazole (Aciphex), omeprazole (Prilosec, Dexilant), and dexlansoprazole (Dexilant).

The sixth proton pump inhibitor consists of a combination of sodium bicarbonate and omeprazole and (Zegerid). All proton pump inhibitors except Zegerid are best used as an hour before meals. This is a critical timing because proton pump inhibitors work best when the production of acid is at a peak in the stomach, and this occurs after meals. When the proton pump inhibitors are used before meals, they will be very active during the production of acid in the stomach after meals. This will make them work well and stop the secretion of acid to prevent GERD.

Pro-motility drugs
Pro-motility drugs are the drugs for GERD, and they work by stimulating the muscles of the gastrointestinal tract (GIT), including the stomach, small intestine, esophagus, and colon. Metoclopramide (Reglan) is one pro-motility drug that is approved for the treatment of GERD. Pro-motility drugs increase the pressure that is present in the lower esophageal sphincter (LES), and they are also known to strengthen the contractions (the peristalsis) of the esophagus. Both of these effects are expected to reduce acid reflux from the stomach. However, these effects that the pro-mobility drugs have on the esophagus and sphincter are small.

Both effects would be. However, these effects on the sphincter and esophagus are small. Consequently, it is assumed that the primary effect of this drug, metoclopramide, may be to increase the rate of emptying of the stomach. This is very important as it would be expected to reduce acid reflux from the stomach.

The best time duration you can use pro-mobility drugs is 30 minutes before meals. They are also retaken at bedtime. Pro-mobility drugs cannot be taken to treat complications or symptoms of acid reflux; they are not just effective in treating them. Therefore, these drugs are either used to boost other treatments for GERD, or they are used for people who do not react to other GERD treatments.

Foam barriers
Foam barriers are those drugs that provide a unique form of foam for the treatment of GERD or acid reflux. Foam barriers are tablets, and they composed of a foaming agent and an antacid. Once taken, the tablet will disintegrate once they reach the stomach. The tablet will turn into foam that will float on the top of the stomach liquid contents, including the acid. The foam creates a physical barrier to prevent the reflux of liquid from reaching the esophagus. At the same time, the antacid that is attached to the foam will have to neutralize any little acid that is trying to escape into the esophagus when they come in contact with the foam.

The best time to take the tablet is after eating, that is when the stomach is distended. It is also recommended that GERD patients should take the tablet when lying down. These are the times when acid reflux is more likely to happen. The foam barrier tablets are not always used as the only or the first drug for treating GERD. They are rather added to other drugs for the treatment of GERD. They can also use them when other GERD drugs are not relieving the patients from the symptoms effectively. The one and the only known foam barrier tablet is a combination of alginate (Gaviscon), magnesium trisilicate, and aluminum hydroxide gel.

GERD surgery

The drugs that we have discussed above are only effective in treating the complications and symptoms of GERD. Sometimes, they are not very effective in the treatment of GERD, and that is why this option is available. For example, even after the successful and sufficient suppression of acid and release from regurgitation, heartburn, with its potential for problems in the lungs, GERD may still occur. However, the number of drugs that are needed most times for the satisfactory treatment of GERD are sometimes so great that they do not worth it again. In a situation like this, the best treatment to resort to is surgery. Surgery is the only solution that can stop the reflux in this situation.

Fundoplication is the surgical procedure that is performed on GERD patients to prevent reflux in them again. This surgery is called anti-reflux surgery or reflux surgery. During fundoplication, the surgeons will have to pull out any hiatal hernia sac that is found, they will take it below the diaphragm, and they will stick it there. In addition to this, they will have to tighten the opening in the diaphragm through which the esophagus passes through into the stomach around the esophagus.

Finally, they will have to wrap the upper part of the stomach that is very close to the opening of the esophagus around the lower esophagus sphincter; they will then create an artificial lower esophageal sphincter. The best way they are doing this surgery is by performing laparotomy (making an incision in the abdomen). Another way is by making use of the technique called laparoscopy. A small viewing device and other surgical tools are passed into the stomach through numerous small puncture sites that are made in the abdomen. Laparoscopy is a procedure that prevents the need for making a major abdominal incision.

Surgery is very effective in treating the complications and relieving symptoms of GERD. Up to 80% of patients of GERD will have excellent relief of their symptoms for up to 10 years. However, many patients with GERD who have had surgery for the treatment will continue to take medications for reflux. The use of these drugs after the surgery is not clear whether they are using it because they are still having reflux and symptoms of reflux, or they are taking it to prevent other problems related to GERD that may arise after the surgery.

One of the most common complications that arise after fundoplication is swallowed foods that got stuck at the artificial sphincter. Luckily, food sticking to this sphincter is usually temporary. If this is becoming permanent, they need to use endoscopic treatment to dilate (or stretch) the artificial sphincter; this usually will relieve the patient from the problem. Occasionally, they do re-operate the patient to revise the prior surgery.

Endoscopy

Very recently, there has been the development of endoscopic techniques for the effective treatment of acid reflux or GERD. This technique has been tested and confirmed. One type of endoscopic treatment, which basically tightens the sphincter, involves stitching (suturing) the part of the lower esophageal sphincter. The second type of endoscopic treatment involves the use of radio-frequency waves to the lower area of the esophagus just directly above the sphincter.

The radio-frequency waves will have to cause damage to the tissue that is beneath the esophageal lining; this will then create fibrosis (or scar). As this scar shrinks, it will be pulling the surrounding tissue to the center of the sphincter, thereby causing the tightening of the sphincter and the part above it.

The third type of endoscopic treatment for acid reflux or GERD involves the injection of resources into the wall of the esophagus in the area around the lower esophageal sphincter. The materials that are injected will tend to increase the pressure in the lower esophageal sphincter and thereby prevent the reflux of the stomach liquid from happening. The injected material in one treatment was a polymer.

Unfortunately, the injection of a polymer material led to the creation of serious complications that lead to the unavailability of the material for injection. In another treatment that was discontinued, they inject expandable pellets into the esophagus of the patient. The third material that is currently in use is gelatinous polymethylmethacrylate microspheres. There is little information about this, so we cannot say whether it is still available or effective.

One advantage of the use of endoscopic treatment for GERD is that it does not require surgery, and it can be accomplished without hospitalization. There is limited experience with the use of endoscopic techniques for the treatment of acid reflux. This shows that we don't know how effective they are when it comes to long term usage. Since we don't know the effectiveness and the type of complications that may come with the treatment, endoscopic treatment should only be done as an experimental trial.

Prevention of transient lower esophageal sphincter relaxation

Transient lower esophageal sphincter relaxations seem to be the most common way that makes the occurrence of acid reflux possible. Although baclofen is a drug that is available for the prevention of relaxations, it has complications that are too recurrent to be useful. Researches are going on for the production of drugs that will prevent lower esophageal sphincter relaxation without having side effects on GERD patients.

What is a rational approach to the management of acid reflux (GERD)?

There are different ways to approach the management and evaluation of acid reflux or GERD. The approach depends on the presence of complications, adequacy of the response to treatment, and the severity and frequency of symptoms. For the most common symptom of acid reflux or GERD, infrequent heartburn, an occasional antacid, and lifestyle changes may be all that is needed to treat it. However, for frequent heartburn, it may be adequate to use daily non-prescription-strength or over-the-counter (OTC) H2 antagonists. You can also use a foam barrier with the H2 antagonist or the antacid.

If a foam barrier, non-prescription H2 antagonists, and life-style changes and antacids do not sufficiently relieve heartburn, it is time to pay a visit to your doctor for further evaluation of the GERD and its symptoms and to consider prescription-strength drugs. Your physician should do an evaluation that will include an assessment for likely complications of acid reflux or GERD. He should base his treatment on the findings such as asthma, sore throat, cough, hoarseness, unexplained lung infections, difficulty swallowing, or anemia (due to ulceration or bleeding from esophageal inflammation). You should also seek clues that may resemble the presence of GERD, such as esophageal motility disorders and duodenal or gastric ulcers.

If the GERD patient does not have any signs of complications or symptoms and no suspicion of other diseases, they should make use of H2 antagonists with a therapeutic trial of acid suppression. However, if H2 antagonists are not sufficiently effective for the treatment, a second trial can be given (it involves the use of the more potent PPIs). Sometimes, the trial treatment could begin with a PPI and avoids or skips the H2 antagonist.

Now, no further evaluation should be necessary if the treatment relieves the symptoms from the patient completely; this case, they will continue using the effective drug, PPI, or H2 antagonist. However, as we have already discussed, all these commonly used approaches come with potential problems; this is why some doctors or physicians will always recommend taking a further evaluation to almost all the patients that they see.

If during the time of evaluation, some signs or symptoms suggest a disease other than GERD or complicated GERD or if the respite of symptoms with PPIs or H2 antagonists is not satisfactory, it will be recommended that they go for further evaluation by endoscopy (EGD).

Since the results from endoscopy come in different ways, there is a different approach to the treatment of each possible result. If the GERD patient has his esophagus to be normal with no other diseases found, the goal of the treatment will be just to relieve the symptoms off the patient. Therefore, prescription-strength PPIs or H2 antagonists are appropriate for the treatment. If there is damage to the esophagus (ulceration or esophagitis), the goal of the treatment will be to provide healing to the damage done by the reflux. In a situation like this, PPIs will be preferred over H2 antagonists; this is because they are more effective when it comes to healing.

If there are complications of GERD like Barrett's esophagus or stricture found in the patient, it is more appropriate to treat such patients with PPIs. However, to get the adequacy of the PPI treatment, the patient should be evaluated with a 24-hour pH test while they are treating with the PPI. Although the quantity of acid reflux to control symptoms of GERD, it may still be unusually high. (Therefore, it is not satisfactory to judge the adequacy of suppression of the acid reflux by just the ability of the patient to respond to treatment.)

They can also treat strictures with the use of endoscopic widening (dilatation) of the esophageal narrowing. They can also do a periodic endoscopic examination to identify the premalignant variations in the esophagus with Barrett's esophagus.

If, after the treatment with maximum doses of PPI, the symptoms of GERD do not respond, there are two different options for management. The first option for management is to perform a 24-hour pH testing to decide whether if the patient is having any disease other than GERD or the PPI is ineffective for the treatment. You may try giving a higher dose of PPI if the PPI is ineffective, and you can treat the other disease if present. For the second option, you just have to increase the dose of PPI and skip the 24-hour pH testing.

In another treatment option, you have to add another medicine to the PPI; the drug should be working in a way that is not similar to that of the PPI. For example, you can add a foam barrier or a pro-motility drug to the PPI. If it is needed, you can add all the three types of drugs just to make sure that the person is treated. If there is no satisfactory response to this treatment (a maximal one indeed) after this, they should perform a 24-hour pH testing.

Now, with the condition above, who should consider an endoscopic treatment trial or surgery for GERD? Since the effectiveness of the recently established endoscopic treatments cannot be guaranteed yet, we cannot suggest this as a better option. However, the patient should be the one to consider surgery if he or she still has regurgitation that cannot be managed with drugs.

Surgery recommendation is critical, especially if the patient's regurgitation results in infections of the lungs. There should also be surgery for those who multiple drugs or large doses of PPI fail to control their reflux. If a patient does not like to take life-long drugs to ease or stop the symptoms of GERD, he or she should go for GERD surgery.

Some surgeons (physicians) recommend that patients with Barrett's esophagus should resolve this problem with surgery. This is to recommend that surgery is believed to be more effective and operational than endoscopic surveillance and abnormal tissue, followed by treatment with drugs (acid-suppressing drugs). There are no research and studies that show the superiority or effectiveness of surgery over ablation or drugs for the treatment of acid reflux and its complications.

What are the unresolved issues in acid reflux (GERD)?

Inconsistent relationships among heartburn, acid reflux, and damage to the esophageal lining (esophagitis and the complications) is one of the unresolved issues in GERD. Others include the following questions that need immediate answers to find a perfect solution to acid reflux and its symptoms and complications:

1. Why is it that not all the episodes of acid reflux that a patient with GERD feels cause heartburn?

2. Why is it that some patients with slightly increased acid reflux suffer from heartburn, and other patients do not even with the same amount of acid reflux?

3. Why do many patients have heartburn in their esophagus even with no signs of visible damage?

4. Why do many people with more damage done to their esophagus have less heartburn than people with little or no damage to their esophagus?

5. Is heartburn related to the absorption of acid across the esophageal lining and not to the inflammation of the esophagus?

All the above questions show that we have a lot to learn about the relationship that is between esophageal damage and acid reflux and about the mechanisms (processes) responsible for heartburn. The issue of heartburn is now of more than passing interest. The knowledge of the processes that produce esophageal damage and heartburn is now raising the possibility of getting new treatments that would help to get a solution to every problem related to acid reflux and acid reflux itself.

One theory that has been proposed to get a solution to the above issues involves the reason behind the pain that people feel when they are suffering from acid refluxes. The researchers believe that the pain and discomfort are caused by stomach acid reaching and making contact with the inflamed esophageal lining. However, the lining of the esophagus is not always inflamed. With this, the acid may be provoking the pain nerves that are located within the esophageal wall behind the lining.

While this may be the correct explanation of the problem, there is another explanation that is backed up by the work of one group of scientists. These scientists were able to find out that heartburn occurred due to the shrinkage or contraction of the muscle in the lower esophagus sphincter. It is confirmed that the contraction of the muscle leads to pain. The contraction could also be known as an epiphenomenon; this means that the refluxed acid causes the muscle to contract when it stimulates pain nerves, but the contraction does not cause the pain. To confirm this, more studies are necessary to make the causes of heartburn is clear.

Importance of non-acidic reflux

Apart from acid, other potentially harmful agents are always refluxed into the esophagus. An example of this is bile. However, it has recently been confirmed that it is difficult or impossible to identify non-acid reflux accurately. Therefore, it is important to study whether the cause of the symptoms is non-acid reflux and whether it is injurious or not.

There is a new technology that determines the presence of non-acid reflux possible and accurate. The technology involves the use of measurement of changes in impedance within the esophagus. This method will be used to detect reflux of liquid. It is possible to identify reflux by adding a pH test to the measurement of impedance to tell whether the reflux is acid or non-acid.

We don't know anything yet about the importance of - acid reflux and whether it is causing symptoms, esophageal damage, or complications. With more studies, we will be able to see this clearly and resolve the problems surrounding non-acid reflux.

The problem with pills

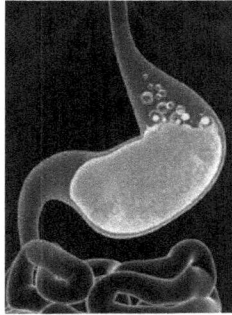

Why do you think there will be problems with pills? Why don't you think that the use of pills will help to neutralize or restrict the production of stomach acid? They do work well, but the problem is that these drugs will not work for a long time and they are not meant for continual use. They can have negative side effects over time.

After continued use of antacids, they can lead to diarrhea or constipation by upsetting the digestive tract. Also, the use of proton pump inhibitors like Prilosec and Prevacid for the reduction of the production of stomach acid has been linked to increasing the risk of pneumonia, osteoporosis (which means brittle bone disease), and negative drug interactions.

Unfortunately, most of the pills available in the market today have done little to get rid of this incident. Approximately 40 % of adult Americans are now suffering from acid reflux. And amazingly, there is now up to 500% in the rate of esophageal cancer in the U.S. since the 1970s. According to a study, it has been shown that up to 9800 GERD victims that were using proton pump inhibitors for treatment have an increased risk of having esophageal cancer.

Natural Remedies

Apart from the use of pills and diets, there are a lot of several other natural treatments that may help you relieve acid reflux or GERD symptoms. Some of these natural remedies include ginger, slippery elm bark, and deglycyrrhized licorice. All of these may reduce symptoms, improve gastric emptying, and it may also relieve nausea.

According to research, it has been confirmed that slippery elm contains high levels of mucilage. Mucilage is an ingredient that can help to coat and soothe the stomach and throat. Mucilage may also help the stomach to improve its secretion of mucus; this helps to protect the stomach from acid damage. It will also prevent the acid from finding its way to the esophagus.

According to research that was done in 2010 in BMC Gastroenterology, it suggests that the use of an oral melatonin supplement for the relieve of the GERD or acid reflux symptoms. Although this is only recommended as part of the treatment, there must be some other form of treatment like having dietary or lifestyle changes or the use of other medication or the use of surgery. All these will help to get rid of acid reflux finally and successfully.

BENEFITS
10 Benefits of Getting Rid of Acid Reflux

A s we have already seen that having acid reflux can make one suffer from many health issues, and its symptoms can be severe most times. However, getting rid of acid reflux will provide more benefits to the patient, and the patient will live a healthy lifestyle again. While some of the benefits of getting rid of acid reflux have to do with the total elimination of reflux symptoms, others are associated with the secondary benefits of getting rid of acid reflux triggers (for instance, you may have to lose weight). All these are very important, and while some benefits impact the quality of life, others impact on physical health. All are important. Below are some of the benefits you can get from getting rid of acid reflux:

1.   A Good Night's Sleep

Unable to sleep is one of the common complaints that we receive from acid reflux patients. They complain that the reflux messes with their sleep and prevents them from having good quality sleep. Acid reflux can be the nemesis of having or getting a good sleep at night, whether it is preventing you from falling asleep or sleeping well, making you uncomfortable, or waking you up.

Many other factors may prevent people from sleeping well; the fact that they eat their largest meal for the day before sleeping at dinner can be one of the important factors that you need to look into. Lying down is another factor to look into. When you lie down, there will be no gravity to help you battle with the reflux from your stomach. This way, the liquid content in your stomach may flow from your stomach into your esophagus. Whatever the cause of your acid reflux, getting rid of it will help you turn bad night's rest into a nightmare.

2.   Better Overall Health

When you have acid reflux, many dietary changes were recommended for the treatment of reflux. This will, in turn, have a positive consequence on your overall health. Many notorious dietary culprits are associated with the treatment of acid reflux – one of them is high-fat food and another one is smoking. The most harmful personal habit is the consumption of high-fat diets. In the United States alone, this contributes to an approximate of 300,000 deaths annually.

Doctors also recommend the reduction of alcohol intake and the overall quitting tobacco as well when you have reflux. Although this may look like punishment to many people suffering from acid reflux, it will help to boost your overall health. Quitting smoking and reducing alcohol intake as part of your acid reflux attack plan will help you reduce your risk of having severe health conditions like cancer and heart disease. This will also help you get rid of your acid reflux totally.

3.   Goodbye Heartburn

Heartburn is the main symptom of acid reflux, and it is associated with pain in the chest. One of the most important benefits of getting rid of acid reflux is the fact that pains in the chest due to the presence of heartburn will be reduced. If you have been battling with pain in your chest, you will see that there is nothing fun about daily discomfort when the pain is done. Chronic pain has become part of the acid reflux package for many people who are battling with acid reflux.

Most of the pains of acid reflux are associated with heartburn, but this pain can also result from other symptoms that are associated with acid reflux. Some of these include an esophageal stricture or a sore throat. Regardless of what causes the pain, chronic pain can affect everything concerning your lifestyle from the physical ability to overall happiness. However, when this pain is no more there, you will be free from pain, and you will be able to do everything easily and without pain.

4.   A Clearer Mind

Getting rid of acid reflux can also help you improve your state of mind; it will also help you with a positive impact on cognitive abilities. The pain and interrupted sleep that is linked with acid reflux can have a philosophical impact on the ability of a person to think and concentrate clearly. Regularly, dealing with acid reflux could affect relationships, grades, or job performance. In addition to this, dealing with the loss of sleep, chronic heartburn, and poor diet and other hallmarks of acid reflux also improve mental abilities. You will have a clear mind when you deal with all of these symptoms of acid reflux and acid reflux itself successfully.

5.   A Brighter Disposition

When you are suffering from acid reflux, not only your mental capabilities will be affected, you will also have a problem with your emotions and attitude. Even the years of insufficient sleep, chronic heartburn, and other complications that are linked with reflux can wear down the brightest disposition you have. When you are exhausted from battling with acid reflux, it will be hard to enjoy life and be happy.

While your mood will be affected, the moods of your loved ones and those around you will be affected too. Once you have one cranky and tired person among you, you should know that it is not easy to deal with one. Reflux can make someone hostile, moody, or even depressed. Once you can treat the person off the acid reflux, you people will be free too. You will not be blamed for being a little grouchy after having a sleepless night of restless tossing and turning or of terrible heartburn.

6.   Getting Reduced Stress

It can be draining to carry the burden of GERD or acid reflux every day and be living with the pain. There is no how good or healthy your body is; the impact of acid reflux will affect your day-to-day activities. Although this problem does not have much impact on what you eat, it also does not affect what you can do and what you cannot do. All of these lead to stress. However, once you can get rid of your acid reflux, you will have no stress to worry about again, and you will be free to move on with your daily life challenges.

7.   Fewer Doctor Visits

Most of the lifestyles that you are practicing and following when you have acid reflux are helpful for your overall health. You will not have to revisit the doctors when you can get rid of acid reflux successfully. A well-balanced diet that you are practicing when there is a problem will provide your body with all the energy and nutrients that it needs. This will give you fewer reasons to avoid paying a visit to the doctor.

8. Stop The Inflammation and Tame the Flame

If you have a chronic sore throat, chronic cough, and asthma, getting rid of acid reflux is particularly important. Although there is no direct link between acid reflux and asthma, yet, there are shreds of evidence that having acid reflux can worsen or trigger asthma attacks. People who are often attacked with sore throats or chronic coughs are often diagnosed with acid reflux. This can mean that there will be a slight relationship between the two. If acid reflux is the reason for your discomfort and inflammation, eliminating or reducing reflux can simply mean that you will be saying goodbye to your sore throat or cough.

9. Reduced Risk for Cancer

By getting rid of acid reflux, you can considerably reduce your risk of developing some severe medical conditions that can affect your life. Barrett's esophagus is one of the most critical issues that is associated with gastroesophageal reflux disease (GERD) and acid reflux. Barrett's esophagus is a condition that affects the tissues and cells lining the esophagus; it makes these cells and tissues worse. Although Barrett's esophagus is a severe condition, it can also lead to the development of another serious condition known as esophageal cancer. This means that once you can get rid of reflux, you will get rid of the chance of getting cancer. For every year you have Barrett's esophagus, the probability of developing esophageal cancer increases.

10.   **Show Me The Money!**

Your wallet is the last place that getting rid of acid reflux will affect. You will see the benefit of living a reflux-free life is in your wallet. This is because battling with acid reflux for a very long will cost a lot of money, and you will be having a reduction in your account. Whether you have to treat your reflux with an occasional antacid or you have to go and buy prescription meds daily, weekly, or monthly, you will surely pay a cost to fight reflux.

Getting rid of acid reflux, its symptoms, and complications are the best thing that a person suffering from it can do. This will make it easier for them to live a normal and perfect life and be free from discomfort and embarrassment. If you have not suffered from it before, you would not know the pain these people go through. The pain is one of the reasons why they must find a lasting solution to this reflux problem. When they are free from the problem, they will enjoy the benefits listed above.

Recipes of plan

Reflux-Free Meal Plan for a Week

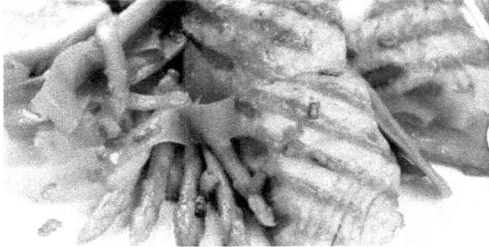

No matter your condition about acid reflux, it is better to get a recipe for the plan for your condition to make you better. Whether you are a new patient who has just been diagnosed with acid reflux or you are a vet who is getting off the track with diet, you may find it challenging to find foods that will work well for your body. According to health professionals, it has been confirmed that people with acid reflux have a great success and a reduction in their symptoms when they avoid common food triggers. Some of these foods that trigger or worsen the acid reflux symptoms include chocolate, onions, high-fat foods, caffeine, tomatoes, and more. This is under the data released by the International Foundation for Gastrointestinal Disorders.

Below is a better recipe for a plan that will offer you a week-long meal plan. This meal plan will provide you with reflux-friendly eating. This tasty idea listed below will help you get back on track in no time. Follow this meal plan for a week, and you will get better in no time. Once you finish the first week, continue with the plan for the next three weeks, and you will be relieved from the problem of acid reflux and its symptoms.

Sunday

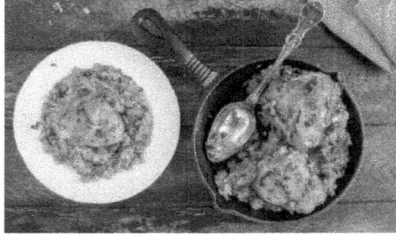

Breakfast: Rice Chex cereal took with almond milk and sliced banana

Breakfast Snack: Sliced apple should be taken with almond butter.

Lunch: You can take tuna salad wrap.

Lunch Snack: Banana bars made with 2 cups oat flour, 2 ripe bananas, 2 eggs, and 1 cup sugar, which is baked at 350 degrees until it's perfectly done.

Dinner: Gluten-free chicken spaghetti, or you can take baked chicken thighs over rice.

Monday

Breakfast: Green smoothie made with mango, coconut milk, spinach, and banana.

Breakfast Snack: Banana bars

Lunch: Peanut butter and honey sandwich with baked potato chips.

Lunch Snack: Dates and almonds.

Dinner: Baked chicken thighs over rice or take turkey and avocado wrap.

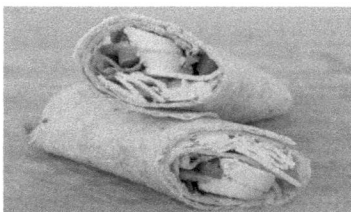

Tuesday

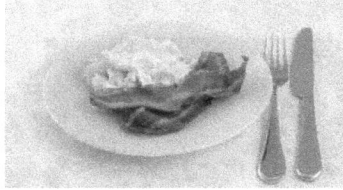

Breakfast: Simple rice pudding made with rice milk, cooked rice, and sugar.

Breakfast Snack: Granola bar

Lunch: Avocado and turkey wrap.

Lunch Snack: Baby carrots and hummus.

Dinner: Homemade shrimp lo-mein made with soy sauce, fresh ginger, and rice noodles. You can also take eggs and turkey bacon.

Wednesday

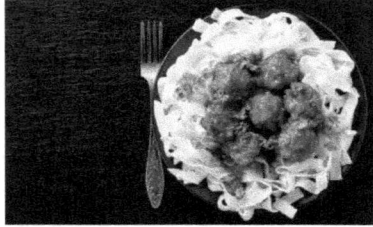

Breakfast: Turkey bacon and eggs.

Breakfast Snack: Banana slices with coconut yogurt.

Lunch: Mixed greens topped with chicken salad.

Lunch Snack: Baked rice crackers.

Dinner: A baked potato with baked pork chops. You can also make gluten-free pasta on turkey meatballs.

Thursday

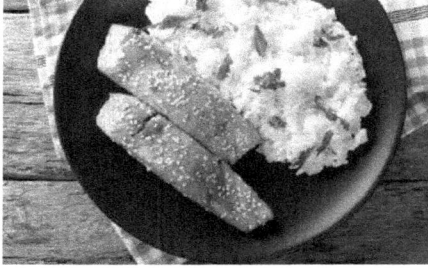

Breakfast: Oatmeal topped with maple syrup and walnuts.

Breakfast Snack: peanut butter placed on rice cakes.

Lunch: Boiled eggs with applesauce and crackers.

Lunch Snack: Air-popped popcorn

Dinner: Gluten-free pasta placed on turkey meatballs (you can make extra meatballs for tomorrow's lunch). You can also eat honey glazed salmon with rice.

Friday

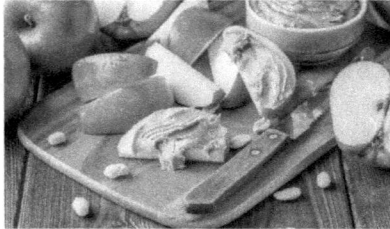

Breakfast: Peanut butter smoothie made with yogurt, peanut butter, milk, and banana.

Breakfast Snack: Trail mix without adding chocolate on top.

Lunch: Meatball sub (do not use tomato sauce but mayonnaise on top of the meatballs).

Lunch Snack: Baked potato chips added with ranch dip.

Dinner: Rice with honey mustard glazed salmon added to it (or you can try salmon patties). You can also take peanut butter and apple slices.

Saturday

Breakfast: Yogurt parfait made with bananas, blueberries, and Greek yogurt.

Breakfast Snack: Peanut butter with sliced apples.

Lunch: Shrimp salad wrap.

Lunch Snack: Gluten-free cookies (you can also try butter shortbread cookies made by Pamela).

Dinner: Homemade pizza made with melted cheese, a gluten-free crust, and sautéed mushrooms.

To get relieved from the symptoms of acid reflux, the meal plan above can be followed for three weeks. Although this is not easy, and it will deprive you of what you like the most, getting a solution to your problem or pain should be of higher priority. Once you can get rid of the acid reflux, its symptoms, and complications, you will be free to eat anything you like. And lastly, these foods are the best for your body because they come with all the necessary nutrients that will be useful to your body.

A meal plan that works well for you when you have chronic heartburn

If you know that you are suffering from chronic heartburn, you must avoid spicy foods. In addition to this, make sure you keep up some dazzle in your diet that includes fresh herbs and low-fat sauces. If you just eat a great meal, the fiery feeling of heartburn will be what will remind you of such a meal. However, you will not want to feel the pain of heartburn again, and that is why you must avoid every worse food that may worsen your heartburn and other symptoms of acid reflux.

However, when your doctor confirms that your gastroesophageal reflux disease (GERD) has led to chronic heartburn, you should be worried about eating a bland and disappointing meal in the future. A gastroenterologist at Massachusetts General Hospital, Dr. Kyle Staller, says that this may not be true anyway because different people have different kinds of food that may trigger their heartburn. What he suggests is that everybody suffering from heartburn should keep a journal with him or her. This will be used to determine and avoid which foods are causing or worsening the symptoms of their acid reflux.

Common culprits
There are a lot of foods and ingredients that may intensify heartburn; some of these include citrus, tomato sauces, spicy foods, and vinegar. You need to avoid all these foods and ingredients if you are used to eating them.

Fatty and fried foods are those foods that stay longer before digestion in the stomach. While they are in the stomach, this may lead to an increase in the stomach pressure, and this may force open the muscles that prevent the stomach acid from reaching the esophagus (the lower esophageal muscle or LES). When this happens, there will be reflux.

Other common heartburn triggers are onions, peppermint, chocolate, caffeine, carbonated drinks, and alcohol. You must try as much as possible to avoid all of them as they may worsen your symptoms of heartburn and acid reflux in general. Although getting rid of or avoiding them is not easy, you have to cure your pain first.

What to eat for dinner?
You can enjoy foods such as poultry, vegetables, legumes, lean meats, fish, fruits, and whole grains for your dinner. The trick here is making them flavorful.

However, if you are disturbed with spices, you can try to use only a small quantity of them in your meal. Also, you must be mindful of blends that contain chili powder and cayenne. You can use fresh herbs instead. This is because fresh herbs may be less irritating because they are less concentrated, says Emily Gelsomin, who is a registered dietitian at Massachusetts General Hospital. What she recommends is the use of oregano, fresh parsley, and basil.

Here is another tip - always roast your food. Roasting of food makes the vegetables sweeter. This is because the natural sugars in the vegetable will come out and caramelize. What works well include sweet potatoes, cauliflower, broccoli, carrots, squash, and Brussels sprouts. Grilling, broiling, or sautéing, of foods will bring out their powerful flavor.

Eat vegetables raw. Since your symptoms may become worse when you eat tomato sauce, you may have to use fresh tomato instead. Fresh tomato may not bother you, and it may not worsen your symptoms, says Gelsomin.

Use sauces but reduce the fat. Always blend low-fat yogurt with sauté mushrooms or cucumber and basil in a little olive oil. You can also make the pesto by blending Parmesan cheese, pine nuts, basil, and a dash of water or olive oil. Use a tablespoon of the pesto on your food before eating; Gelsomin suggests this.

Breakfast and lunch
For your breakfast, avoid eating fatty meats like bacon or ham. Oatmeal is a great option in this case. You can also throw in raisins, bananas, and maybe a hint of cinnamon to your breakfast suggests Gelsomin. There are several other possibilities, including low-fat yogurt with nuts or fruit, whole-grain toast, any eggs, or a side of chilled whole grains such as quinoa that is topped with a splotch of yogurt or mixed with fruit.

For your lunch, think of eating salads with protein such as beans or chicken. However, to avoid vinegar and citrus, think of using a yogurt-based dressing, says Gelsomin.

How to avoid heartburn

Heartburn is another name given to acid reflux or gastroesophageal reflux (GERD). It is called heartburn because it makes your chest feels like it is on fire, burning, says the MD, and a gastroenterologist at the University of Missouri Health Care, Matthew Bechtold. When people feel like they have a burning sensation in their chest, they use the word "heartburn" to describe it. This is really refluxed of acid from the stomach into your esophagus that is happening and causing the chest pain.

However, according to Dr. Bechtold, he says that this is not just a burning sensation, but it is a feeling that the food in your stomach is coming back up into their esophagus or throat. It also feels like you have a chronic cough; this happens especially at night when you are lying down flat. Due to the inflammation in the esophagus, you may also have trouble swallowing.

There are a few reasons as to why this happens. According to Dr. Bechtold, he says that some foods trigger the reflux of liquid from the stomach into the esophagus. This is possible because those foods will help to relax the lower esophageal sphincter (LES), making it easier for the liquid contents to pass through the esophagus. Those foods are trifecta, also known as "three big sins" because they contain chocolate, caffeine, and alcohol, especially red wine.

When any of these is present in food or drinks, they will relax the LES (lower esophageal sphincter) muscle, thereby allowing acid from the stomach to come back up. Rudolph Bedford, a gastroenterologist doctor from Santa Monica Health Center in California, explains that adding acidic foods (such as citrus fruits) and spicy foods (such as tomatoes) to foods can worsen heartburn as they are also common perpetrators.

Fortunately, there are also a lot of foods that will help you combat heartburn by either helping to relieve it or preventing it from happening. Here are some of the foods you might want to consider adding to your meal to help relieve you of the burn.

Oatmeal - Yes, oatmeal is a kind of boring food, but it is a good food choice for relieving people from heartburn. It is recommended that eating oatmeal for breakfast helps to prevent heartburn. For you to have a reflux-free day, you can wake up to a bowl of easily-digested oats. Oat will not worsen your heartburn because it will prevent acid reflux from your stomach from reaching your esophagus.

Ginger – Dr. Bedford recommended the use of ginger as dietary management and treatment for heartburn. It is known that ginger has a long history of medicinal use, and it helps in dissolving digestive issues. Most of us have once used ginger ale to get rid of an upset stomach. No matter how you want it - chewed on like candies, steeped in hot water for tea, or grated or sliced fresh into recipes - you can incorporate ginger into your meal.

Aloe Vera – We all know that aloe vera is good for our skin when it is sunburned. However, have you ever wondered if it will help you fight acid reflux? You can drink aloe vera juice to relieve yourself from the pain of acid reflux. Many patients have found the use of aloe vera very helpful to them. While many people blend up aloe juice or smoothies to drink at home, you can save effort and time by grabbing the pre-made aloe vera from most health food stores.

Banana – To get your recommended servings of fruit per day, you can incorporate bananas into your diet. Bananas are a smart and low-acid choice for people who are suffering from acid reflux. Banana is cheap and readily available; they help to relieve the symptoms of acid reflux. You can eat it by adding some sliced banana on top of your oatmeal.

Melon - Melons are also low in acid, just like bananas, according to Dr. Bedford. You have to reach out for cantaloupe or honeydew instead of going for other fruit staples such as oranges or grapefruits, which could worsen your already-sensitive tummy.

Turkey and chicken - Put down that large, fatty steak! You should choose lean meat options such as 90/10 ground beef, turkey, and chicken without the skin. All these are very important for your acid reflux symptoms, and they will help prevent your chest from having a feeling of being on fire!

Fish and seafood – When it comes to having reflux-friendly seafood, there are a lot of options out there for you, including lobster, clams, shrimp, fillet of sole. However, there are a lot of options available for the cooking of this seafood - you can sauté, grill, or bake it. The only cooking method that you should not do with seafood is to fry it. This is because the grease could just worsen your heartburn. The best alternative is for you to toss shellfish with little whole wheat pasta. You can also get a bed of brown rice and lay a few ounces of fish on it for a yummy meal. Such a meal will prevent you from feeling the burn.

Parsley – If you are looking for a remedy for your heartburn, you can plant some parsley in your garden today. Just like ginger, parsley can soothe an ailing stomach and prevent acid reflux to your esophagus. You can mix parsley into smoothies or recipes, or you can chew on a few of the parsley leaves whenever the reflux strikes.

Bread is also a better option that goes easy on the esophagus, and it is not likely to worsen or cause any discomfort to you. To make it healthier, you can go for a heart-whole grain option to increase the fiber content. Do you like avocado? You are in luck! Healthy fats that those that are in avocado are better and they are likely to cause or worsen your heartburn than those that are found in queso, French fries, and bacon. If you must eat fats, add healthy fats like reflux-friendly seeds, nuts, and eggs to your diet.

Since eating more veggies can help resolve a few health problems, it is not a surprise that they work well for heartburn too. This is because vegetables like leafy greens, carrots, and peas are so low in sugar and fats.

They don't have much in them that could worsen your reflux symptoms. You can also add a salad to your meals; they are your friends.

Diet and Lifestyle Changes

The best way to get rid of acid reflux is by changing your lifestyle. Changing of lifestyle is by making changes and modifying things that we can control. Lifestyle changes involve factors that may bring changes to the symptoms of reflux or make them worse. Some of these include changes in daily routine or dietary changes. Although diet does not cause acid reflux, gastroesophageal reflux disease (GERD), and its most frequent symptom or complaint of heartburn, these can be aggravated by the type of foods we are eating. In addition to diets, many medications can aggravate symptoms. If you are using any type of medication before or during your battle with reflux, make sure you disclose the medications to your physician.

The burning sensation that you feel in the chest right behind your breastbone is heartburn. This is a condition that we feel when we start to see the presence of stomach acid in the esophagus (food tube). There are a lot of things that you have to change and start doing when you have this symptom. Once you start doing this, you will be relieved from the pain of the symptoms. Some of what you can do (in terms of diet and lifestyle) to get rid of or relieve yourself from the pain of heartburn or acid reflux are as follows.

Position

One of the best things that play an important role in the control of reflux is gravity. To explain this, you need to observe the fact that your food may come back to your esophagus, especially when you have less than normal lower esophageal sphincter (LES). If this happens, you may experience food in your esophagus, and this will cause heartburn. Once you start experiencing heartburn, you will start feeling pain in your chest. This usually happens when you lie in bed at night, and it occurs after meals, or after taking a nap after a meal. To prevent heartburn, you need to maintain an upright posture or a sitting position for some hours until your meal is fully digested.

However, if you are feeling reflux or heartburn regularly at night, you must look for a solution. The best solution to prevent heartburn from occurring at night is by inserting a triangular wedge to keep the upper part of your body higher or by raising the head of your bed. This will help you keep your esophagus higher than your stomach. Avoid performing exercises after a meal. This is because exercises contract the abdominal muscles. This contraction can force food through a weakened esophageal sphincter. Maintaining a standing or sitting position until the meal is digested will help you prevent heartburn. This is especially true of exercises that involve bending, such as cleaning the floor or lifting.

Tip – Never lie down within three hours of eating a meal. This is because three hours after a meal is the time when acid production is at a peak in the stomach. So plan and take your dinners early and avoid taking bedtime snacks.

How you eat

Have you thought that how you eat can affect your condition with reflux? How you eat is much more important than what you eat. If you decide to eat a large meal, you will be exerting more pressure on the lower esophageal sphincter. When you take a snack at bedtime, it will be positioned in a way that reflux will be easy when you lie down. The best thing to do is to eat early in the evening, like three hours before thinking of going to sleep.

This way, the food will be digested before sleeping. The recommended eating pattern is by eating the main meal at noon and eating a very light food late in the evening as dinner. You should always eat your meal in relaxed, stress-free surroundings. You should suspend going to the kitchen to fetch food or minding children and the performance of any other tasks until after the meal. To minimize reflux, you should take smaller meals in an upright, relaxed posture.

Tip – Avoid taking large meals, particularly late in the evening as dinner before going to bed. Try to make your main meal your lunch or as the mid-day meal.

What you eat

There are a lot of foods that trigger the ability of the lower esophageal sphincter to prevent reflux. These foods are best avoided in the evening during lunchtime or before lying down or exertion. These types of meals differ from person to person. Some of the common foods that trigger reflux include onions, fats, and chocolate; they are particularly troublesome. Commonly, alcohol provokes heartburn, and it does this by compromising the lower esophageal sphincter, stimulating stomach acid production, and by irritating the esophagus.

Common beverages such as tomato juice, tea, cola, citrus juice, and coffee (both caffeinated and decaffeinated) may worsen symptoms. They do this by stimulating stomach acid production and by irritating the esophagus. Many other foods may bother some people; these people should discover the food that triggers their symptoms and avoid or reduce eating those foods. This is for their benefit.

Tip – Experiment to find the type of food that does affect and does not affect you. You should start by eliminating or reducing onions, fatty foods, and chocolate.

Many other oral medications can trigger the symptoms of acid reflux if they are allowed to rest in the esophagus. Some of these medications include the antibiotic tetracycline and potassium supplements. To be on a safer side, you must always swallow medication while in an upright position. Also, don't forget to drink lots of water after swallowing the medication.

Other factors

There are other factors that can aggravate reflux. Being overweight can stimulate reflux. This is because having excessive fats in your abdomen can put more pressure on the stomach. To prevent this, you need to find a way to lose a moderate amount of weight. Also, heartburn is affected by pregnancy, especially in the first three months. This is possible because certain hormones will be weakening the lower esophageal sphincter. In addition to this, having a crowded abdomen encourages reflux. Generally, the absence of too much weight leads to the improvement of heartburn after delivery. Lastly, strong emotion and stress can also influence heartburn.

Detailed food lists and easy to understand explanations

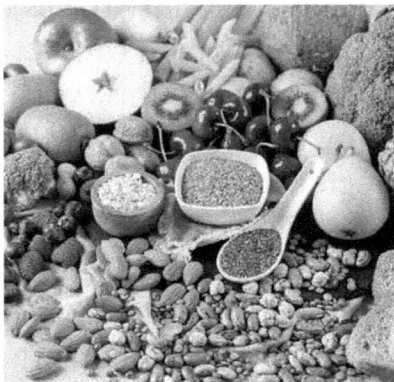

Diet Restrictions and Nutrition Guidelines for People with Acid Reflux

Acid reflux or gastroesophageal reflux disease (GERD) is a type of digestive disorder that causes liquid from the stomach to reflux or flow back up into the esophagus, thereby causing problems. This type of backflow is known as acid reflux. This reflux is known to occur when there is a malfunction in the lower esophageal sphincter (LES). The lower esophageal sphincter is the ring of muscles that are found between the stomach and the esophagus. The work of these muscles is to allow easy passage of liquid and food into the stomach; the muscle will open to allow food and liquid passage, and it will close back to prevent the flow of liquid from

144

the stomach into the esophagus. However, in people with GERD, this muscle will become weak, and they work irregularly because they relax and contract abnormally. This abnormal contraction and relaxation of these muscles lead to the flow of stomach contents and acid to move into the throat and esophagus.

Acid reflux often causes irritation and discomfort in the esophagus, and this often leads to having a bitter or sour taste in the mouth and throat. This is usually followed by a burning sensation in the chest (this is also known as heartburn). Some other people who are suffering from acid reflux also experience sore throat, dry mouth, nausea, coughing, and other uncomfortable symptoms.

When there is prolonged acid reflux to the esophagus, there is bound to be inflammation in the esophagus, and this will lead to a condition that is called esophagitis. This condition may make it difficult and painful for the person to swallow food. When this is left untreated, acid reflux can cause damages to the esophageal lining and lead to esophageal irritation and ulcers. When this happens, the person may start to experience narrowing of the esophagus, bleeding, or Barrett's esophagus, which is a condition that causes the cells that are lining the esophagus to change and look like those found in the intestine. This can simply mean that there is a growth of esophageal cancer.

Currently, there are many medical cures and treatments for acid reflux; changing diets is one of the most affordable and the easiest ways to manage symptoms. Diets can also help to prevent acid reflux from improving and from happening in the first place.

What Makes a GERD-Friendly Diet?

There are a lot of foods that are very hard to digest, and they can lead to an increase in the production of acid in the stomach. Once this occurs, there will be the presence of acid reflux into the esophagus and the presence of other acid reflux symptoms. Although there is no common food that can trigger acid reflux in every patient, there are different food that triggers these symptoms from one person to another. However, the common food that triggers acid reflux is high-fat foods, alcohol, and spicy foods. Another important thing to notice is to avoid every food and drink that you know that cause discomfort to you when taken. This also helps to integrate foods that can prevent or ease acid reflux symptoms.

List of foods to avoid entirely

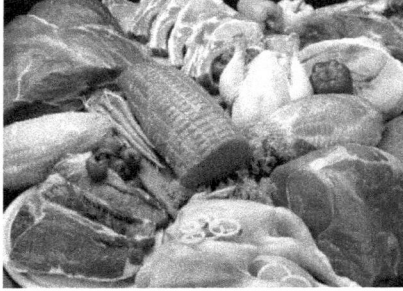

One of the best ways to avoid experiencing heartburn and acid reflux is by avoiding taking large meals. This is because large meals will cause enlargement of the stomach, thereby making it easier for the acid to flow into the esophagus. To get this right, it is important that you take five to six small meals per day and not just two or three large ones. In addition to this, you mustn't eat food for at least three hours before going to bed. Although what triggers acid reflux varies from one person to another, make sure you avoid garlic, mints, onions, fried foods, spicy foods, soda, and other carbonated beverages during your meals. These beverages and foods are known to aggravate acid reflux symptoms because they can trigger reflux from your stomach.

What to limit

There are a lot of foods you can eat when you are suffering from acid reflux, but the problem is that you must eat them in moderation. This type of food may cause discomfort when eaten in large quantities, and the degree of discomfort varies from one person to another. Here are some beverages and foods that may trigger acid reflux symptoms. With this, they must be consumed in small quantities.

Beverages - mint tea, tomato-based drinks, citrus juices, alcoholic beverages, regular and decaf coffee, and whole milk or chocolate milk. These beverages have a higher acid content that may aggravate the acid in the stomach already.

Fats - gravies, cream, margarine, and butter. This is because they stay longer in the stomach than any other food type, and this may increase the pressure in your stomach, thereby making it easy for stomach liquid to reach your esophagus.

Carbohydrates - French fries, potato chips, doughnuts, croissants, tortilla chips, and plates of pasta prepared with creamy sauces or pesto.

Fruits and Vegetables - fried vegetables, tomatoes, citrus fruits, such as lemons, oranges, and grapefruit, and vegetables prepared with cream sauces.

Protein - fried fish, sausage, fried meat, pepperoni, bacon, hot dogs, and fried chicken.

Desserts - ice cream, chocolate, and pies, high-fat cakes, and cookies.

What to include in your diet?

As you can see, it may seem that there are a lot of delicious foods that you must not eat or eat in small quantities because you are suffering from acid reflux, but actually, there are a lot of foods you can eat. There are a lot of GERD-friendly foods that will not cause you any problem when you eat them every day. This means that you can consume these foods without causing triggers to your acid reflux. The goal of this is to provide meals that have all the necessary nutrients that will be healthy for your body. Such healthy food will include complex carbohydrates, lean protein, and fruits and vegetables. Below are some of the foods you need to incorporate into your daily meals.

Beverages - non-mint herbal teas, nonfat or low-fat milk, and non-citrus juices.

Carbohydrates - crackers, waffles, boiled potatoes, tortillas, pancakes, whole-grain bread, low-fat cereals, rice, plain pasta, oatmeal, and low-fat muffins.

Fruits and Vegetables - non-citrus fruits, such as melons, bananas, and apples, and all vegetables with little added sauces or fat.

Protein - tofu, eggs, peanut butter, beans, peas, lentils, low-fat cheese, low-fat yogurt, and lean meat, such as chicken and fish.
Healthier Fats - low-fat salad dressings, low-fat mayonnaise, nuts and seeds, and small amounts of sesame, vegetable, olive, and sunflower oils.

Desserts - sponge cake, frozen yogurt, hard candy, low-fat ice cream, angel food cake, sherbet, and low-fat cookies.

When you start eating the right food for your acid reflux condition, it does not mean that you will stop the consumption of all your favorite foods. The best way this will not affect your current diet is by just making a little change to it and the way you eat it. This will help to prevent or ease the symptoms of GERD. One last thing you can do if the symptoms of acid reflux do not change when you change your diet and another lifestyle, you need to schedule an appointment with your physician or doctor. To know the severity of your condition and to determine the type of treatment that best suits you, you need to let your doctor perform various tests on you.

Different ways to get relieved acid reflux or GERD without medication
Before resorting to the use of drugs, there are different lifestyles that you can modify that will help you get relieved from gastro-esophageal reflux. Apart from helping to reduce the symptoms, it can also help you control the acid reflux without spending on drugs. This is one of the ways that your doctor will recommend to you even before he or she starts to prescribe drugs to you.

If you have a sore throat and you sound a little hoarse, it might be that you are about to get attacked by the flu or bracing for a cold. This is a normal feeling that anybody can feel. However, if you have had these symptoms for a while, it may not be that you have contracted a virus, it may just be the actions of a valve in your body, the lower esophageal sphincter. The lower esophageal sphincter is the muscle that is controlling the passage between the stomach and the esophagus. When this passage does not close properly or completely, there is a higher chance that stomach food, acid, and liquid will flow back into the esophagus. This process is known medically as gastroesophageal reflux; when there is a backward flow of the acid from the stomach, it is called acid reflux.

However, many symptoms come with acid reflux. When acid reflux happens, it can cause hoarseness and sore throats, and this may let you have bad taste in your mouth. Once the symptoms of this acid reflux become chronic, it is called gastroesophageal reflux disorder, or GERD. The symptom of GERD that is commonly known to the people is heartburn. Heartburn is a pain in the chest and the upper abdomen. When this pain happens, it can make people feel like they have a heart attack sometimes.

According to an associate professor of medicine and a gastroenterologist at Harvard Medical School and the producer of "A Woman's Guide to Having a Healthy Stomach", says Dr. Jacqueline Wolf, he said that there are three conditions that contribute to acid reflux - delayed stomach emptying, too much acid in the stomach, and poor clearance of acid or food from the esophagus.

If you have been having or experiencing different symptoms of acid reflux or repeated episodes of heartburn, below are some of the ways to get relieved from the pain without the use of drugs:

1. Sleep on an incline

As a person suffering from acid reflux, you should be able to sleep on an incline. Normally, you should sleep with your head about 6 to 8 inches raised or higher than your feet. This can be made possible by making use of "extra-tall" bed risers. This will help to raise the head of your bed, thereby making your head higher than your leg when sleeping. To change your sleeping pattern to this form, you can use a foam wedge to support your head or the upper part of your body. Please do not create wedge support for the upper part of your head by stacking pillows. This will not give you the uniform support you need.

2. Eat sparingly and slowly

There is a higher probability that you will experience more reflux into the esophagus when your stomach is full. You have to prevent having a full stomach by breaking down your meals into smaller sections. You have to try something that is sometimes called "grazing." This is what they used to describe preventing or not eating three large meals daily but frequently eating small meals. This will prevent having a full stomach, and you will be satisfied.

3. Avoid certain foods

The advice that is given to everybody suffering from acid reflux is that they should eliminate from their diets all but the blandest foods. However, according to Dr. Wolf, he says that we are no longer in the days when they forbid us from eating what we love and anything we like. He said that is no longer the case. However, he said that there are still foods that are more like triggers to acid reflux and they must be eliminated.

Some of these foods include tea, chocolate, spicy foods, tomatoes, mint, fatty foods, onions, garlic, coffee, and alcohol. If these foods are taken regularly by a patient of acid reflux, the symptoms might be severe. You must try to eliminate them to see if they help control your reflux. Eliminating them one after the other will let you know which one triggers your acid reflux more than the other.

4. Check your medications

Check the type of medication you are using if they can also enhance your acid reflux symptoms. This is because medications like anti-inflammatory painkillers, tricyclic antidepressants, and postmenopausal estrogen can relax the lower esophageal sphincter. Also, other medications of bisphosphonates like risedronate (Actonel), alendronate (Fosamax), or ibandronate (Boniva), which are taken to boost bone density, can trigger acid reflux by irritating the esophagus.

5. Don't drink carbonated beverages

Drinking carbonated beverages will make you burp. Once you burp, there will be the migration of acid into the esophagus and this will cause your acid reflux to worsen. Instead, you should make sure that you are drinking flat water and not sparkling water.

6. Stay up after eating

Gravity helps to prevent or reduce acid reflux from your stomach. This means that when you are sitting or standing, gravity will help push the food down and keeps the acid where it belongs in the stomach. Stay sited or upright for up to three hours after eating before you go to bed. In other words, you should not take naps after lunch, and you should not take midnight snacks or late suppers.

7. Don't move too fast

After eating, do everything slowly and make sure that you avoid energetic exercise for up to three hours. You can take a stroll after dinner, but performing a more strenuous workout will send acid into your esophagus especially if the exercise involves bending over.

8. Lose weight if it is advised

When you gain more weight, you will be spreading the muscular structure that is supporting the lower esophageal sphincter. This will thereby decrease the pressure that is holding the sphincter closed. Once the lower esophageal sphincter cannot close well, it will lead to having reflux and heartburn.

9. If you smoke, quit

People suffering from acid reflux shouldn't smoke. You need to quit smoking if you want your acid reflux symptoms to reduce. This is because nicotine may prevent the lower esophageal sphincter from contracting; it may relax. Once the lower esophageal sphincter relaxes, there will be reflux of the acid content into your esophagus.

The above are tips that you need to follow if you are suffering from acid reflux. All these will make your life easier and live freely without getting affected by the symptoms of acid reflux. Follow them accordingly and make sure you contact your doctor for advice and more information on how to manage yourself.

Meal Planning Tips to Avoid Heartburn

Are you one of the 15 million Americans that is suffering from heartburn every day? Heartburn is one of the main complications of acid reflux that many Americans are experiencing. The best way to prevent heartburn is by avoiding certain beverages and food. Although this may seem discouraging, it is the best way to prevent heartburn from affecting you. Getting relieved from heartburn has something to do with the size and timing of your meals; this is according to the American College of Gastroenterology. This is why it is imperative to plan your meals well. However, before planning your meals, you must know about heartburn and what causes it.

Why Heartburn Happens

There may be weaker lower esophageal sphincter muscle (LES), or it may be relaxing too frequently in people with frequent heartburn. This gives room for stomach acids to move into the esophagus easily. Heartburns happen when the stomach acid comes in contact with the lining of the esophagus; thereby producing a burning pain in the middle of the chest and injuring the esophagus. Meal planning can be used to halt heartburn.

Tips to Prevent Heartburn
If you are suffering from frequent or occasional heartburn, you can decrease the tendency of relaxing the lower esophageal sphincter with the use of some tips. You can also decrease the probability of the stomach acid (and other stomach contents) from splashing up toward the lower esophageal sphincter by keeping the following tips in mind:

Avoid going to bed for two to three hours after a meal. This is because it will be physically easier for stomach acid to splash and move up to the lower esophageal sphincter when you lie down. Gravity helps to maintain the position of the stomach contents (they will be at the bottom of the stomach) when you sit down or stand up.

Avoid taking foods and drinks that weaken the lower esophageal sphincter muscle like peppermint, caffeine, chocolate, alcohol, and fatty foods. You should also avoid taking beverages and foods that may irritate a damaged lining of the esophagus like tomatoes and tomato juice, citrus and citrus juice, and black pepper and chili pepper.

Avoid eating large meals, especially before going to bed because the stomach content will flow up to the esophagus when the volume in the stomach is increased. You should try taking small meals like four to five times than taking two or three large meals.

Avoid taking high-fat meals because they stay much longer in the stomach because they are not easily digested. Also, fried or greasy foods may weaken the lower esophageal sphincter muscle.

Avoid alcohol and avoid smoking before, during, or after meals. Both smoking and alcohol drinking can weaken the lower esophageal sphincter muscle, and they can result in heartburn.

Avoid exercising immediately after meals; try to wait for at least two to three hours after a meal before exercising if you must exercise. If your heartburn always gets worse after exercise, avoid doing exercise.

Chew a non-peppermint flavor gum after meals to increase peristalsis (the easy movement of food into the stomach and from the stomach into the small intestine) and to improve the production of saliva (for the production of bicarbonate that helps in the neutralization of acid).

Plan your mealtime to boost slow but sure weight loss, especially if you are overweight. This is most important because having extra weight around the midsection can increase the pressure that is going up to the lower esophageal sphincter by pressing against the stomach.

At the end of meals, make sure you drink a small glass of water to help dilute and wash down the meal and any other stomach acid that may be present at the esophagus. This is suggested by the MD of Kansas Medical Clinic, Shekhar Challa.

Plan on heartburn-friendly beverages such as decaffeinated tea, non-fat or low-fat milk, mineral water, water, and non-citrus juices.

Beverages that you must avoid taking when you are suffering from heartburn include:

Juices - Citrus juices and tomato and can irritate an injured esophagus.

Sodas - Sodas can bloat the abdomen, thereby increasing the pressure that you have in your stomach and giving room for stomach acid and liquid to splash up into the esophagus. This will be leading to increased heartburn.

Coffee (even decaf), cola, alcoholic beverages, and caffeinated tea can boost the amount of acid content that is in the stomach in addition to the lower esophageal sphincter.

Eat a meal that is in high fiber. It has been confirmed from a recent study that people who eat and make use of a high-fiber meal plan have less than 20 % probability of suffering from acid reflux symptoms. This does not depend on body weight. Some of the foods that are high in fiber include vegetables, beans, whole grains, fruits, nuts and seeds (mainly unprocessed plant foods).

A Day Sample Menu for Heartburn

You may find it difficult to make use of the tips above without a physical meal example that will help you. Here is a day sample meal that will help relieve you of the heartburn. See how this might work well for you.

Breakfast - Less fat turkey bacon, apple juice, and high-fiber cold or hot cereal with non-fat or 1% low-fat milk.

Morning Snack - 1/2 cup fresh fruit, decaf green tea, and one container low-fat yogurt.

Lunch - Avocado sandwich and roasted turkey on whole-wheat bread. Baby carrots or other raw veggies. Make sure you finish the lunch with a glass of water and chew some non-peppermint gum after eating.

Afternoon Snack - Apple slices, decaf green tea, whole-grain crackers, and reduced-fat cheese.

The above is a sample menu for heartburn. You can use this sample to create your daily menu. See the weekly menu we have above for more information about how to set up your daily meal.

Evening Exercise - Perform easy exercise like three hours after your lunch. This will help prevent acid reflux during bending, especially if you will be performing strenuous exercises, which is not advisable.

Contact your doctor for more information about the type of exercise you should be doing if you must do it.

Dinner (moderate-sized portions of) - Steamed vegetables and Barilla Plus (or any other high fiber pasta) with pesto sauce or less-fat Alfredo sauce with some fish or meat if desired (like strips of lean beef or cooked shrimp). These foods mean that you are not going to eat full because eating full will increase the pressure in your stomach, thereby leading to easy reflux of the liquid from your stomach to your esophagus.

A light dessert (like a frozen fruit bar). Make sure you chew non-peppermint gum after eating and end the food with a glass of water. Chewing gum will stimulate the secretion of saliva, which will help to wash down the acids in the esophagus. The bicarbonate that is present in the saliva will also neutralize the little acid content in the esophagus.

Heartburn Triggers
This is the last thing that you must not fail to recognize. Although you can avoid some, you cannot avoid many other triggers. Some of these triggers include pregnancy, lying down after a meal, alcohol and carbonated beverages, coffee, and tea, eating a large, especially fatty meal, smoking, chocolate, peppermint, tomato sauces (spaghetti and pizza), excess weight, and blood pressure medicines and some muscle relaxers. However, for those you cannot avoid, make sure you visit your doctor for more information and

treatment you need to receive. This will help relieve you from the symptoms and complications of acid reflux.

The Best and Worst Foods to Watch Out for When You Have Acid Reflux

A gassy bloating in the stomach, a bitter taste in the throat, and a hot burning in the chest are some of the symptoms of acid reflux - this is no picnic. How you eat and what you eat are all that contributes to the effect of the acid reflux in your body; they all have an impact. The worst and the best foods you can use for acid reflux could help differentiate between sour misery and sweet relief.

What Aggravates Acid Reflux?

There can be the occurrence of acid reflux when the lower esophageal sphincter (sphincter located at the base of the esophagus) is not working well. This gives room for the liquid from the stomach to flow up into the esophagus. While the best foods for acid reflux can soothe it, other worst foods can exacerbate painful symptoms - says Leena Khaitan. According to Dr. Khaitan, a gastrointestinal surgeon, changes in the diet can affect acid reflux significantly and prevent the effects of other treatments. You need to eat well, and this will make it easy for other medication to work well for you.

Best Foods for Acid Reflux

According to Dr. Khaitan, he says that a diet that is well-balanced with protein, vegetables, and fruits is the best diet for the treatment of acid reflux. When these foods are taken, your reflux will not become worse, and you will be feeling better. Example of such food include:

Chicken breast - Make sure that you get rid of the fatty skin. Choose broiled, baked, or grilled chicken breast and skip the fried one. This will help soothe or relieve your acid reflux symptoms.

Celery, lettuce, and sweet peppers - These mild green veggies are very smooth on the stomach, and they will not cause painful gas that may lead to the reflux of the liquid content from the stomach.

Brown rice - This is a complex carbohydrate that is mild and filling. Please make sure that you do not serve it fried.

Melons - Cantaloupe, watermelon, and honeydew are all low-acid fruits. They are among the best foods that you can eat when you have acid reflux.

Oatmeal - This is a filling, hearty, and healthy food to eat. This is a comforting breakfast, and it also works well for lunch.

Fennel - This is a -crunchy acid vegetable that is very good for acid reflux patients. It has a natural soothing effect, and it has a mild licorice flavor.

Ginger - Chew on low-sugar dried ginger or steep caffeine-free ginger tea for a natural tummy tamer. Always try to use ginger in your meals.

Worst Foods for Reflux

Generally, all GERD patients should avoid anything acidic, fatty, or highly caffeinated. These foods are very worse for reflux, and they must not be taken when the symptoms persist. Below are some of the worst foods for acid reflux:

Tea and coffee - Caffeinated beverages aggravate acid reflux. You should always go for caffeine-free teas. Although caffeine may be sweet, you will forget the sweetness once your acid reflux symptoms started showing.

Carbonated beverages - When you drink these beverages, their will bubbles will expand in your stomach, thereby creating more pressure and pain. To prevent this, choose caffeine-free iced tea or plain water.

Chocolate - Chocolate consist of a combination of three different ingredients that are worse for acid reflux. These include caffeine, fat, and cocoa. The fat stays longer in the stomach and caffeine, and cocoa can help increase the pressure in your stomach. The increase in pressure will increase the risk of getting liquid reflux from the stomach.

Peppermint - Peppermint is an acid reflux trigger. You should not let its reputation for soothing the tummy fool you. Although peppermint is perfect, it is worse for acid reflux.

Grapefruit and orange – Citrus fruits consist of a high level of acid, and it worsens the symptoms of acid reflux because they relax the lower esophagus sphincter. The acid that is present in citrus fruits will increase the acid in your stomach, and it will increase the rate at which you will get reflux and its symptoms.

Tomatoes - Also avoid tomato soup, marinara sauce, and ketchup - they are all naturally high in acid. The quantity of acid they have will start to irritate the esophagus and stimulate the stomach acid to join.

Alcohol - The effect of alcohol on the body is a double whammy effect. Apart from the fact that it stimulates the secretion of acid in the stomach, it also automatically relaxes the valve of the lower esophageal sphincter. Once the lower esophageal sphincter is relaxed, it will give the stomach liquid content easy accessibility to the esophagus.

Fried foods – Fried foods are some of the worst foods for acid reflux. This is not good for those suffering from acid reflux because they may contain an amount of fat and smoke, which will stimulate the enlargement of the lower esophageal sphincter.

Skip the onion rings, French fries, and fried chicken. You can cook in the oven or on the grill at home. Fried chicken and fried foods, in general, is worse for acid reflux or GERD.

Late-night snacks - Avoid eating anything (whether snacks or real meal) in the two to three hours before you lie down or go to bed. Also, you must try to eat four to five smaller meals all through the day instead of eating two to three large meals per day.

Why Don't You Talk to Your Doctor About Your Acid Reflux?

No matter how you are feeling with your reflux, it is highly recommended that you speak with your doctor. This is very important, especially the best foods for reflux do not relieve your reflux symptoms. Your doctor will recommend other alternatives like medication that can block the flow of acid from the stomach, lifestyle changes, and surgical procedures to tighten your esophagus sphincter. If you have acid reflux or heartburn, it is recommended that you make a doctor's appointment. This is important especially if the reflux is frequent or severe.

Also, the Chronic acid reflux, which is known as gastroesophageal reflux disease (GERD), can lead to the growth of esophageal cancer. Visiting the doctor will make it easy for the doctor to recommend the right meal that will work for you. If it is above the use of meal treatment or changes in your lifestyle, the doctor will use the opportunity to diagnose you and decide on the type of medication that you can use to relieve you of the acid reflux symptoms. If this does not work too, the doctor will then arrange how to perform surgery on you.

In summary, if you are feeling some of the symptoms of GERD and acid reflux, you need to visit your doctor, especially if you are developing a burning sensation in your chest or stomach after eating a certain meal. Some of the other symptoms that you may be having include dry cough, burping or hiccups, sore throat, a lump in the throat, difficulty swallowing, and bloating. The earlier you find a solution to your problem, the better it is for you.

Chapter 1 – Heartburn: An Overview

The first step to solving any problem is understanding it, and acid reflux is no different, so that is where we are going to begin.

Most people with heartburn realize they have heartburn, but few people actually realize it goes beyond that. So many people make a list of the foods they can't have, and resign themselves to a life of eating foods they like, but not foods they love.

They remember the days when they were able to have pizza and spaghetti, sausage and bacon, and anything else that they craved without fear that it was going to come back to bite them later on.

I'm sure you remember those days. The days when you went out with friends And indulged in all of the buffalo wings you could hold. You ate jalapenos by the dozen, and didn't bat an eye when the waiter brought out a second round of the chili cheese fries.

You could hold your own with the best in the crowd, tossing back your favorite spicy foods like they were going out of style. You didn't give much thought to anything you were eating, because it didn't matter.

Until that dreadful day.

Heartburn can set in at any time, you don't have to be any certain age, and you it doesn't necessarily matter

the kind of lifestyle you live. More than 3 million new cases show up around the globe every year

Let's take a second to dive deeper into this topic, and pick out some of the major points about it.

Acid reflux: what is it?

At the top of your stomach there is a valve with a special muscle around it. This muscle, known as the lower esophageal sphincter opens and closes as food is passed down to the stomach.

But, when it stops working properly, it can start to open too much or not close entirely when the food has passed into the stomach. The result is that stomach acid creeps up into the esophagus, burning as it does.

Stomach acid, as you know, aids in digestion. The main function of this acid is to break down food, so naturally it erodes anything it touches, which can even be the lining of your esophagus. Don't worry, your body is constantly working to heal itself, so you aren't in danger of anything happening, but you are going to feel that killer burning pain.

What causes it?

While heartburn can strike anyone, there are certain factors that do put you more at risk. Take a look at this list, and see if anything sounds familiar:

- Eating too much or going to bed too soon after eating

- Being overweight
- Eating too much then lying down or bending over immediately after
- Eating too much of certain kinds of foods such as citrus, onions, spicy foods, or fatty foods
- Drinking alcohol
- Taking too many pain relievers or blood thinners

Now do take note that this is not an exhaustive list, and there are other things that could contribute to this problem, but overall, these are the main culprits of this condition.

What are the symptoms?

In general, the symptoms are painfully obvious. There is little doubt that you have heartburn due to the fact your chest feels as though it is on fire. But, that's not the only one.

More symptoms of the disease include:

- Bloating
- Regurgitating or vomiting foods
- Tasting a horribly bitter taste in the back of your throat
- Hiccups that can also burn
- Diarrhea
- Nausea

- Dry cough, wheezing, a sore throat, hoarseness

- Weight gain for no known reason

And again, that's just a rough list.

Thankfully, heartburn is an incredibly easy condition to treat, even if you are having the most severe symptoms. In the chapters to come, I am going to show you what doctors don't want you to know, as well as how you can treat this entirely at home without any synthetic medication.

Don't worry.

Relief is on the way.

Chapter 2 – The Secret Your Doctor Won't Tell You

Most people who have acid reflux know that they have it before they ever go to the doctor. Some people still think you need to go in and get a medical professional's advice, but in all honesty, you can easily diagnose this at home.

Of course, if you are really worried about anything with your health, by all means head to the doctor straightaway, but if you are merely feeling heartburn, odds are you can both diagnose and treat it right in your own home, without ever having to set foot in a doctor's office.

How is it diagnosed?

If you do go to the doctor, you can expect him to run several tests on you.

These tests require you to swallow a special kind of solution that will allow the doctors to see what's going on inside of you with an x-ray, or you can get a device implanted in your esophagus for a couple of days to check the amount of acid you have in it.

Then there's the method in which the doctor sticks a long camera down your throat to see what's going on down there, or a biopsy of tissue taken from your esophagus can show whether or not you have acid reflux.

171

Now, if you read through those paragraphs, odds are they didn't sound like a lot of fun for you. This is no surprise because, well, they aren't any fun. They are uncomfortable, they are cumbersome, and they are, in fact, unnecessary.

If you are feeling the symptoms of acid reflux, especially more than once a week, you can very accurately diagnose this disease within yourself, no cameras, x-rays, or solutions necessary.

The fact is, this condition is so common you can almost always diagnose it yourself with minimal effort, and you can always treat it yourself without ever setting foot inside a doctor's office

Of course they aren't going to tell you this, or they would be right out of a job. But, with a little bit of knowledge on your end, you can not only diagnose yourself with this disease, but you can treat it with entirely natural remedies.

Nothing synthetic, no harmful side effects to watch out for, and no money or time spent at a doctor. You can read what you need, then head out to the store this afternoon to get it, and be well on your way to being healed tonight. With some consistent treatment, you are going to see the symptoms disappear altogether, and this entire bout is going to be a thing of the past.

But, you have to follow the directions, and you have to stick with it. Yes, this is effective, and yes, it is going to work for you, but if you don't follow the directions, or if you try to skip steps, then you are going to be stuck in the same situation you are in now.

Let's break out of the line of conventional thinking and dive into the world of natural remedies. They have been around for thousands of years, and with good reason...they work.

You know how you feel, you know you want to feel better, and you know the solution is right within arm's reach. Let's take the next step now and stop talking about it and actually do it. You are going to be so glad you did.

Your stomach will thank you.

Chapter 3 – The Foolproof Guide To Natural Remedies

In your ques to use natural remedies to treat your acid reflux, you are going to run into all kinds of people with all kinds of opinions.

There are going to be those that say it's not going to work. There's going to be those that are highly supportive and want to know exactly what you are doing to make it work for you, and there are going to be those that say it's going to work for a while, but it's not going to cure your problem.

At the end of the day, what really matters is what you think of it, and how you feel. If you think it's working, keep at it regardless of what other people are saying. You are the only one who knows for sure how you feel, and if you are happy with the results, then keep doing what you are doing.

The key to being successful in treating your acid reflux with all natural remedies is to know *how* to treat something naturally

Of course, when you are taking synthetic medication all you have to do is toss it back and go about your day. But, when you are treating something naturally, it's going to take more effort than that.

Entirely worth it let me assure you, but still, it will take the work.

For most things in life, you aren't going to get that immediate cure we all wish we could have. Yes, there are certainly things you can do or take that will ease the pain if you have a sudden flare up, and there are things that you can do that will start helping you immediately, but overall, curing acid reflux naturally is going to be a lifestyle change.

With that being said, there are many, many small changes you can make to your day that will have a major impact on your day. None of that"all or nothing"kind of thinking allowed here, you have to be willing to make a few small changes, and your problem will be solved.

What are those changes?

Let me show you:

Number 1. Regain balance in your system

Part of the reason you are having issues is because your system is out of balance with itself. If you want to solve your heartburn, you need to get back in sync with yourself.

Try swapping out inexpensive table salt for Himalayan Sea salt. Not only does this taste better, but it's going to help immensely with your acid reflux.

Try adding in a plant based Betaine supplement before you eat a meal, too. It's not much, but the drastic change it makes is going to be well worth it, I promise.

Number 2. Make those necessary dietary changes you need to be making

Most of us will admit that we should be eating better. We should eat more veggies and less junk, and we should cut out the excess fats and carbs and stick with what is healthy.

In all honesty, you don't need to make any drastic changes to your diet, but you really should consider cutting out as many processed foods as you can. You may find some foods aggravate your reflux more than others, but at the end of the day, it's the processed foods that are the real culprits.

Number 3. Help out your digestive system

There are always ways you can help your body function, and some of those things you can do my merely changing out cooked foods for raw. Instead of always cooking your veggies, make sure to eat at least half of them raw.

Make sure you add in plenty of fruits. Real, unprocessed fruits right out of the produce section.

Number 4. Make friends with ACV

To anyone with acid reflux, the idea of adding more acid in on top of what you are already dealing sounds like a terrible thing, but trust me on this. If you add mix a splash of lemon juice with a splash of apple cider vinegar with a small glass of water before each meal, you are going to see a drastic improvement in your acid reflux.

Number 5. Don't forget about that base

In addition to taking ACV, try adding baking soda into your diet regularly. Take note that this could put you at risk for higher blood pressure, so if you are already dealing with this then you may want to skip this method, or you risk changing one issue for another.

If you do decide to take it, you are going to mix a small spoonful in a glass of water, and drink while it still fizzes. Do this once a day, and your acid reflux is going to subside drastically.

Number 6. Bring in that light touch

I can't tell you enough how many good things aloe vera does for you. You can find organic aloe vera at nearly every health food store, and even a lot of department stores.

Mixing in a little bit of this incredibly juice is going to change your life. Not only are you going to feel a lot better, but you are going to see many other ailments you are facing disappear as well. There's no end to the ways you can use aloe in your day, and acid reflux relief is just one of the many countless benefits you are going to see!

Try any one of these remedies, or mix and match to find what really works for you. The entire point of natural remedies is that you have the freedom to find what works for you, even if you are the only person it works for

Now, it's not just the remedies themselves that are important, but you have to also time using them the right way. If you merely try one in the morning, you aren't going to get nearly the same results as you will if you use them throughout your day.

All in all, your day is going to look like this:

Morning: eat something first thing, and follow with a mix of ACV

Mid morning: mix baking soda with water and drink it

Before dinner: drink another round of ACV, but mix less ACV in this time around

After dinner/sometime in the evening: mix an aloe shot and drink that

This doesn't have to be your day every single day, but you do need to roughly stick to a schedule if you want to get the maximum benefits of using natural remedies to cure your acid reflux.

Take the time to learn what works best for you, and stick with that. The more you mess around with remedies, the more you are going to learn what works and what doesn't. Soon, you are going to get in your own system, and your heartburn is going to subside.

Chapter 4 – Immediate Relief For Strong, Sudden Attacks

Overall, when you change your diet and make the little changes in your lifestyle as I listed, you are going to find your life changes drastically. You are going to feel a lot better, you aren't going to have as many attacks, and you are going to be able to eat more foods that you like.

But, as with any condition or disease, there are going to be some days that are worse than others. You may go for days without any symptoms at all, then suddenly get hit with an attack out of the blue.

This doesn't mean you are doing it wrong, and it doesn't mean your treatment isn't working. Your body isn't perfect, just like the rest of the world, so there are going to be times when you just have attacks in spite of your best efforts not to.

What's important isn't that you are having these attacks, it's what you do about your attacks. If you are ready for them when they happen, you will be able to ward them off soon after, making them go away all together.

Try these top three instant remedies whenever you are dealing with the symptoms of acid reflux. The worse the attacks you have, the more you use these remedies

Remedy number 1. Baking soda

Now, I'm not talking about the little bit you mix in your water and drink before a meal, I mean you put an entire spoonful in your water and you chug it as quickly as you can. It's not going to taste that great, but it's going to do the trick.

Again, as I mentioned in the previous chapter, you do need to keep an eye on your sodium intake, and if you do this often you are going to raise your blood pressure. If you already have high blood pressure, you need to be extremely careful with this remedy...only use it in the worst cases.

Remedy number 2. Lemon juice

I like to use lemon juice because it not only makes ACV and baking soda more palatable, but it also helps with attacks that hit out of the blue. As with the baking soda, mix a generous amount with water and drink.

You need to do this as soon as you feel an attack coming on, and wait a second. If the attack doesn't get any better, repeat the steps.

¼cup lemon juice to 1 cup water. Drink.

Remedy number 3. Honey

I could spend an entire chapter explaining all of the benefits of honey alone, and acid reflux remedy is just one on the list. If you feel an attack coming on, or if you feel like you could get an attack, hop right on the honey.

Mix 2 tablespoons in warm water, and drink quickly. I prefer to heat the honey a little so it mixes in better and goes down smoother, but you can do as you please with this. Some people I know prefer to take the honey without water, because letting the honey coat their throat helps.

However you decide to do it, you are going to get better benefits than anything you could ask for if you were using synthetic medication, and you don't have to deal with any of the nasty side effects that go along with them.

As I already said, you can mix and match as you please to get the results you want. Some people prefer doing it one way, some people prefer doing it another. What works for you is what works for you, so discover what that is, and go with that.

Don't be afraid to mix and match some of the remedies and solutions with others. Of course you can't mix the ACV with baking soda, but you can mix it with honey, or you can mix the honey with baking soda.

You can combine the milder remedies found in the last chapter with these stronger remedies you find here to get the kind of results you want. It doesn't matter how you go about it, as long as you are getting the relief you need.

These are all the remedies that you can use for active cases of heartburn and acid reflux. In the next chapter, we are going to look at the specific dietary changes you can make that will keep you from having to deal with this again in the future

After all, prevention is the best cure.

Chapter 5 – Prevention Is The Cure: Lifestyle Tips To Prevent Further Heartburn Flares

You could make a career out of treating your acid reflux, always chasing the one thing that is going to work all the time, every time. Of course, you are going to find as soon as you switch to these all natural remedies that you aren't going to have to deal with the symptoms nearly as often, but there are still dietary changes you can make that will aid in your overall quality of life.

In this chapter, I am going to show you exactly what you can do to maintain a healthy lifestyle and not have to deal with heartburn nearly as often, or as badly if it does come up.

First things first:

When you are trying to make any kind of dietary changes, it is important that you keep a food journal. This will not only keep you on track with what you are supposed to be eating, but it will also help you see what foods trigger the worst symptoms.

Write down what you eat, and how you feel after you do. If you eat something consistently and you feel great, add it to the list of foods you can have without a thought to them. If you eat something consistently and it makes you have symptoms, make a note of how you need to use a remedy while you consume the food.

Avoid the high fat and highly processed foods

In general, we should stay away from the processed foods anyway. There is little nutrition to be found there, and a lot more cons that outweigh any convenience they allegedly bring.

The foods I am talking about include:

- French fries
- Fast food
- Prepackaged foods
- Full fat dairy products
- Pork (primarily bacon)
- High fat desserts such as ice cream and others like this

In addition, you are more likely to have symptoms if you consistently eat these kinds of foods, so make sure you have both your remedies on hand, and that you moderate these foods as much as possible.

Watch the citrus

There are a ton of benefits that come from consuming citrus on a regular basis. But, anyone with acid reflux can tell you that citrus is one of the worst things for symptoms.

It seems the tomato has no sooner than hit your stomach than you are bent over feeling as though you are going to die.

No one wants to feel that way, and it's always best to not chance things. On the other hand, it can be hard to give up certain foods that contain tomato products, so you have to choose.

I recommend you limit your intake of citrus and tomatoes, but you don't have to get rid of them all together. If you are going to consume something with tomatoes or citrus, make sure you use one or two remedies at the same time.

The more you remember to use the remedies, and the more you use them on time and properly, the more you are going to be able to have the foods you enjoy. You may still encounter some symptoms, but overall, you are going to find that the remedies help a lot.

The less often you eat these kinds of foods, the less they are going to be able to cause you problems, too.

Keep the extras in moderation

When it comes to such things as spices, you have a lot more control. More often than not it's the hot spices that cause the most problems, and more often than not you have complete say over if those are in the dish or not.

The best way to handle this is to use things in moderation. Of course, keep using your remedies along with each meal you consume with spices in it and you won't have an issue, but at the same time, make sure you are watching your intake of these foods.

You have a ton of control over the foods you put in your body, so make good use of that control and keep the trigger foods at bay. I want you to be able to eat anything you like, and that includes the foods on the list that can cause issues.

If you live a life where you tell yourself that"you can't"have certain foods, it is only a matter of time before you cave in and over indulge. You need to learn how to use these things in moderation, and combine this use with the remedies I have outlined for you in the previous chapters.

Read through the list of remedies, and head to the store. Always have AVC on hand, and make sure you have your aloe vera within reach, too

Find your preferred remedies, and keep them on hand for when the symptoms appear. As I have said, the more you make this lifestyle a habit, the less often you are going to have these symptoms to deal with...but, as with anything, you are still going to have days where you do feel sick.

The goal of this book is to give you options. The option to prevent it as much as possible, and the option to treat it in the way that you want when it does come up. This is going to take some time, and you will have to work at it to learn what works best for you, but as you learn, you will feel better and better.

Acid reflux is a nuisance, but it's something you can control. With minimal, consistent effort, you are going to gain control of your life back, and enjoy the complete freedom you deserve to have.

Conclusion

There you have it, everything you need to know about acid reflux, and how you can take care of it for good. You know you have spent enough of your life trying to find relief in things that don't give you what you need.

The tips and tricks you find in this book are easy to understand, easy to follow, and just what you need to kick the acid reflux problem for good. You can rest easy knowing that your heartburn is going to be gone, no matter what you eat or what time of day it is.

I hope this book was able to inspire you to take control of your life once more. I hope you follow the directions I have outlined, and you get the results you are want. I hope you kick the disease to the curb and enjoy life like you once did.

This book is everything you need to make that happen, and with the simply directions you have found, you will be back on track and back to your old self in no time at all. Say goodbye to the reflux and pain, and hello to your old life once more.

You deserve to live a healthy and happy life. One that you can live without any pain in your chest. This book provides what you need to make that happen, so get out there and be your best self again.

www.ingramcontent.com/pod-product-compliance
Lightning Source LLC
Chambersburg PA
CBHW060324030426
42336CB00011B/1197